D0831635

TAI CHI

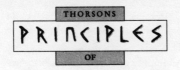

THORSONS
PRINCIPLES
OF

TAI CHI

PAUL BRECHER

Thorsons
An Imprint of HarperCollins*Publishers*

Thorsons
An Imprint of HarperCollins*Publishers*
77–85 Fulham Palace Road,
Hammersmith, London W6 8JB

Published by Thorsons 1997
1 3 5 7 9 10 8 6 4 2

A catalogue record for this book
is available from the British Library

ISBN 0 7225 3474 4

Text illustrations by Peter Cox

Printed and bound in Great Britain by
Caledonian International Book Manufacturing Ltd, Glasgow

THIS BOOK IS DEDICATED
TO THE LOVE OF MY LIFE,
MY WIFE ALEXANDRA.

CONTENTS

ACKNOWLEDGEMENTS

I would like to thank
Peter Simon, Jamie Catto
and especially Nic Alderton and Christina Digby
for their help with the editing of this book.

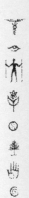

FOREWORD

I met Paul Brecher some years back when he visited me here in Australia as part of a 'searching out' worldwide tour.

He was then, and is now, a genuine young man with a passion for his Taijiquan. I showed Paul the Old Yang Style of Taijiquan (Tai Chi Chuan) and from then onwards he was hooked on this explosive form which is unlike any other Taijiquan.

Over the years, Paul studied hard and attended every workshop that I gave in London. He also visited me here in Australia from time to time to train.

Now, he has written an excellent book on Taijiquan. You will discover in this book things that have not been written about Taijiquan before, simply because the other authors have not known about the older style of Taijiquan. For many years my voice rang out clear but not many noticed. Nowadays the Old Yang Style of Taijiquan is well recognized but not many outside the World Taiji Boxing Association know how to perform or teach this style.

Paul has presented a well thought out work on the principles of Taijiquan for both beginners and advanced students of the art, no matter what style they practise.

Having read this book, the reader will probably wish to get in touch with a teacher of this style of Taijiquan. Nowadays, luckily, we have many such teachers all around the world, including Paul Brecher in London.

This book will add a new dimension to your Taijiquan and internal martial arts training and will grace a good place on your bookshelf.

Erle Montaigue
Master Degree China
World Chief of the World Taiji Boxing Association

GENERAL INFORMATION ABOUT TAI CHI

This book is for all those who are interested in developing their understanding of and ability in Tai Chi, whether they are new to the subject or have been practising for many years.

It covers the theoretical, philosophical and historical sides of Tai Chi, as well as the practical principles, to help readers gain further benefits from their training, and understand Tai Chi not just intellectually but through their personal experiences.

Later chapters in the book go into detail about how to practise Tai Chi correctly. This first section answers the ten most often asked questions about Tai Chi.

WHAT IS TAI CHI?

Tai Chi is a Chinese martial art, originally used for self-defence. Today most people practise it for the great health benefits it has to offer, and for self- and spiritual development.

The book covers these aspects equally because they all enhance and balance each other out. For example, for a weak person to have good self-defence skills, he needs to be healthier and stronger. A person who wants better health needs to develop a more positive attitude because the mind influences the body. And for the person who is trying to become more spiritual, practising Tai Chi for self-defence helps to keep them grounded in the real world so that they don't get lost in the clouds.

The central part of any Tai Chi system is the *form*. This is a single person, an empty-handed series of continuous, smooth, circular, flowing movements. Some forms contain a few movements and can be done in a few minutes, others contain many movements and can take over half an hour to complete.

Tai Chi also has many two-person sparring systems, such as *Pushing Hands*, *Da Lu* and *Lung Har Chuan* (Tai Chi Dragon Prawn Boxing). The *Old Yang* style of Tai Chi has a two-person fighting form called the *San Sau* which is very forceful and invigorating. The *New Yang* style of Tai Chi has a simplified version of the San Sau which is more gentle.

Tai Chi also has weapons forms, such as the *Sword and Dagger*, the *Single Sabre* and *Double Sabre*, the *Short Stick*, the *Staff* and the *Spear*. There is also a *Walking Stick* form which is becoming very popular.

Some styles of Tai Chi contain explosive movements called *Fa Jing*. *Fa* means to release and *Jing* is internal force; so Fa Jing are sudden explosive releases of internal force.

Tai Chi is sometimes referred to as a *soft* style. *Soft* means that during training there is no tension in the muscles or mind. This allows for greater ease of movement and an increase in the circulation of blood and energy around the body, which in turn produces a state of relaxation and calm. These aspects of Tai Chi have made it attractive to many people as a type of stress release exercise.

Some people mistakenly think that *soft* means the movements are feeble and the attitude passive. On the contrary, the movements are dynamic and resilient, and the attitude is one of confidence and decisiveness. This positive attitude builds self-confidence and has also been shown to boost the immune system. Building a strong fighting spirit into the self-defence aspects of Tai Chi also boosts the immune system.

For many years in the West there was a conception that Tai Chi was for the old or infirm, but now it is realized that people of all ages can benefit. If training starts at a young age, it can prevent illness from developing.

Tai Chi is sometimes called an *internal* style: it is not just a form of physical exercise but also a type of Chi Kung. Chi Kung means 'exercises that generate and circulate Chi energy around the body by following certain principles of posture, movement and breathing'.

For your Tai Chi to be a true internal style you need to incorporate into your training the Ten Points of Correct Tai Chi Posture, the Ten Internal Principles of Tai Chi and the Ten Methods of Practice of Tai Chi, all of which are explained in detail later on in this book (*see chapters 2, 3 and 4*).

WHAT DOES TAI CHI MEAN?

Tai Chi is an abbreviation of Tai Chi Chuan. There is no single translation for these Chinese words; they carry many philosophical and poetical meanings as well as literal ones.

Tai Chi is the name of the Yin Yang symbol below:

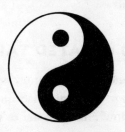

4   *Chuan* means fist, but implies martial art. So together Tai Chi Chuan means the 'Yin Yang fighting system'.

Tai Chi contains closed-fist punches, open-hand techniques, kicks, locks and throws. An experienced martial artist can recognize these moves in their Tai Chi forms, but many people upon seeing the relaxed smooth and flowing movements of Tai Chi for the first time cannot believe that they have anything to do with a martial art.

The main aim of the Yin Yang theory is to attain a dynamic balance in all things at all levels. Tai Chi balances your energy, which connects with both the mind and the body, harmonizing them both.

When they practise Tai Chi, people with poor health become stronger, and those with a tendency to be hyperactive become more at ease. People who feel anxious become more confident, and those who have an angry temperament feel calmer. Eventually Tai Chi produces a happy, healing feeling in everyone. For this reason Tai Chi Chuan is also translated as 'The Way of Supreme Harmony'. You do not have to be Buddhist, Taoist, or of any particular religion or race to gain from the practice of Tai Chi.

Tai Chi should not be confused with *Chi*, which by itself means 'life force energy'; and *Jing*, which means 'internal force', should not be confused with *Ching*, which means 'vital essence' (hormones).

In this book, I have shortened Tai Chi Chuan to the more familiar term Tai Chi.

WHO CREATED TAI CHI?

Scholars cross-reference ancient manuscripts and come up with lists of names and dates; martial artists quote oral histories that have been handed down from master to student for hundreds of years; and in martial arts folklore there are stories of revelations in dreams and of movements being taken from watching snakes and cranes fighting.

A combination of the above will be closer to the truth but ultimately there is no definitive answer to this question.

AN ANCIENT SYSTEM

Records exist indicating that as far back as the eighth century a martial art similar to Tai Chi was practised in China. It was developed by Hu Xuan Ming who was from An Huei province and lived on Tse Yang Mountain. His system was called *Three Generations and Seven*; it was an internal style with many similar techniques and ideas to Tai Chi.

Around this time another Tai Chi-like system called *Hsien Tien Chuan* was created by Li Tao Tze, but little is known about its form and content.

In the 10th century, Liang Kon Yu created the *Nine Little Heavens* system which is very similar to Tai Chi.

These are a few of the documented examples which show us that styles similar to Tai Chi have been around for over a thousand years.

CHANG SAN FENG

The majority of researchers regard the originator of Tai Chi to be Chang San Feng, who lived some time between the 12th and 15th centuries. He spent ten years learning healing methods and martial arts from the fighting monks of the Buddhist Shaolin Temple, then at least another ten years learning more varieties from the Taoist hermits who lived on Wudang Mountain. He is said to have created Tai Chi by combining the best principles of the martial arts styles and self-healing techniques he had learnt.

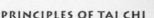

Chang Sang Fen was a great healer who taught others his Tai Chi system because he wanted everyone to have the opportunity to gain from its great health benefits. He was also a great fighter and is reputed to have killed over one hundred people in hand to hand combat.

He reached an incredibly high level of ability and lived to be over a hundred years old. Legends say that he did not die, but transformed himself into pure spirit and flew away.

Chang wrote down some of his methods, which have been handed down from generation to generation and today form part of *The Classics of Tai Chi*. Here is my translation of an extract from his works:

The body must move as a single unit
at one with the breath, Chi and Spirit.

The rooting of the feet, the strength of the legs
and the power of the waist all manifest in the hands.

There is Connection within the whole body.
Our movement is guided by our Intention.

Tai Chi is like a great river rolling on unceasingly.

WANG TSUNG YUEH

A more recent possible creator of Tai Chi was Wang Tsung Yueh who lived in the 18th century. He wrote down his methods which have also become part of *The Classics*. Here are some extracts (my translation):

Yin and Yang continually transform within each move,
without this balance we are double-weighted.

Allow the Chi to gather in the Lower Tan Tien,*
from long practice develop Jing.

Pursue the opponent and move as he moves,
know his intention whilst concealing yours.

To be an unequalled fighter results from this.

* The Lower Tan Tien is a major energy centre located just below and behind the navel. The Middle Tan Tien is located behind the solar plexus and the Upper Tan Tien behind the point between the eyebrows. Although the Middle and Upper Tan Tiens are used in advanced Tai Chi, for the first few years beginners concentrate on the Lower Tan Tien, so that they develop a low centre of gravity, mental balance and stability.

Although many styles are practised, the three main branches of Tai Chi that exist today are the *Chen*, the *Yang*, and the *Wu*.

1. THE CHEN STYLE

Wang Tsung Yueh taught Tai Chi to Chiang Fa, who, some say, taught it to the Chen family. The Chen family say it was one of their own ancestors, Chen Wang Ting, who created Tai Chi in the 17th century. Chen Chang Xing (1771–1853) inherited the system, and it was his great-grandson Chen Fake (1887–1957) who brought the Chen family style of Tai Chi to Beijing and public attention in 1928.

We will never know for sure how it got there, but Tai Chi is still practised in the Chen family village in Henan province. The Shaolin Temple is relatively close to the Chen family village and may well have influenced the Chen style.

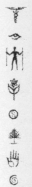

↻. THE YANG STYLE

The story of Yang Lu Chan (1799–1872) is hard to verify. After completing his training in the Shaolin Temples fighting systems, he learnt Tai Chi from a group of martial artists who lived on Wudang Mountain. This group's lineage went all the way back to Chang Sang Feng.

Yang Lu Chan formulated his own version of Tai Chi which is today called the Old Yang style. (This is because his name was Yang; it has nothing to do with Yin and Yang.)

He then set out to find a better fighter than himself. Whenever he heard of a martial artist in the area he was passing through he would challenge them. Often he fought with several people at once but he was never beaten.

He visited the Chen family village and, after defeating some of their best fighters, explained some of his theories to them which they incorporated into their family style to make it into Tai Chi.

Another account says the Chen family fighters were defeated only because Yang was using skills he had learnt from them at an earlier time.

We will never know the truth. Today some people say the Yang style comes from the Chen style and others say they influenced each other, but they are clearly different styles.

Eventually Yang's reputation was so great that when he arrived in Beijing he was asked to be Instructor of the Royal Guard and became known as 'Yang of No Equal'.

Yang Lu Chan taught his Old Yang style to his son Yang Jian Hou (1839–1917) and his grandson Yang Shao Hu (1862–1930), who taught it to his second cousin Chang Yiu Chun, who taught it to my own teacher, Erle Montaigue.

Probably the most widely practised style of Tai Chi today is the simplified New Yang style, developed by Yang Lu Chan's other grandson, Yang Chen Fu (1883–1936).

Yang Chen Fu's most important students were Chen Wei Ming, who wrote the first books on Tai Chi for him, and Tung Ying Chieh, who created *Tung's Fast Form*. His other important students were Tien Sou Lin, who appears in Yang's book, and his eldest son Yang Sau Chung, who died in May 1985. All these people, including Chang Yiu Chun and Yang Shou Hou, appear in a famous photograph taken in 1929.

Cheng Man Ching was not one of Yang Chen Fu's main students and only pushed hands with him on two occasions. His name was never written down in Yang Chen Fu's class diary. He only trained with Yang Chen Fu for about six months learning the basic version of his simplified form. From this he created an even simpler and much shorter form known as the *New Yang Style Short Form*.

Cheng Man Ching publicized Tai Chi in the USA, so he and his form are now familiar to many people.

3 · THE WU STYLE

The second most widely practised style is probably the *Wu* style, developed by Wu Chien Chuan (1870–1942). He learnt from Wu Quan You (1834–1902), who learnt from Yang Pan Hou (1837–1892), the brother of Yang Jiang Hou.

A less well known *Wu* style was created by Wu Yu Hsiang (1812–1880). He was a student of Yang Lu Chan and Chen Ching Ping, so his style was born out of a combination of the Yang and Chen family styles.

Wu Yu Hsiang's style was passed on to Hao Weizheng (1849–1920) and Sun Luctang (1861–1932). Only a few people today practise the *Sun* and *Hao* styles of Tai Chi.

Wu Yu Hsiang contributed to *The Classics of Tai Chi*. Here is my translation of some of his writings:

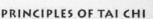

The body follows the Chi which follows the Intention,
If the movement is Sung (relaxed) we develop the Jing.

Jing is generated in the spine like drawing a bow,
Fa Jing is like the release of an arrow.

Our form is dynamic like a falcon about to seize a rabbit,
Our Spirit is sharp like a cat about to catch a rat.

Be as stable as a mountain and flow like a river.

ANIMAL QUALITIES

Animals are frequently mentioned in *The Classics of Tai Chi*, and referred to in the names of many Tai Chi movements, for example: *The Crane Cools its Wings, Monkey Strike, Snake Spitting Venom, Grasping the Sparrow's Tail*, and *Draw the Bow to Shoot the Tiger*. The movements have the characteristics of the animals, and certain animals have qualities that Tai Chi practitioners want to develop: your health and self-defence would benefit if you had the strong bones of a tiger, the vision of a bird of prey and the lightning speed of a striking snake. All Tai Chi movements are similar to those of a snake; the whole body rotates and twists continuously.

If you stand on one leg in a Tai Chi posture, you should have the strength, balance and stability of a stork, and your hands should move like the wings of a bird. In self-defence, your impact with the opponent should have the same force as a bird of prey impacting with the quarry at the end of its power dive.

Your steps should be taken like a cat, which feels the ground before it puts its foot down. Your level of attentiveness should be like that of a cat about to pounce on a mouse, coiled and ready to spring. As soon as the cat senses that the mouse is about to move, it pounces, claws extended and back arched as it makes the offensive movement. In Tai Chi, you do the same: extend your fingers and arch your back as you attack.

Cats lie down with their tails touching their noses. This behaviour shows the universal nature of the internal Chi Kung exercise known as the *Small Circulation of Chi* (*see chapter 5*).

Both Tai Chi and Chi Kung draw some of their knowledge from the observation of wild animals. But mostly, they have developed through the observation of people.

HOW DOES TAI CHI WORK?

Tai Chi heals the body by encouraging Chi (life force) to flow through the acupuncture meridians. Chi connects the mind and body with each other and the world. It is what the strands of 'the web of life' are made of.

The acupuncture meridians run through the entire body, connecting every part. They are different from the nerves, blood, and lymphatic vessels, but they influence these and other body systems because they run through them all.

In a 1991 report by the World Health Organisation, over four hundred acupoints and 20 meridians (the Twelve Organ meridians plus the Eight Extra meridians) are discussed. These acupoints are the points at which the meridians can be accessed.

In the same year, Western scientists verified the existence of the meridians by using a Superconducting Quantum Interference Device to map the lines of the force fields of electromagnetic energy generated by the human body. They were found to correspond exactly with the acupuncture meridians documented by the Chinese over two and a half thousand years ago.

In children, the acupuncture meridians are usually open and the flow of Chi through them is strong. This gives them the energy to run around for hours and hours, and to laugh and cry without inhibition.

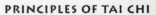

With age, the flow of Chi through the channels can be impaired by mental and physical tensions, poor diet, unhealthy lifestyle and illness.

When Tai Chi is practised daily, the flow of Chi through all the acupuncture meridians can be increased, and health and vitality regained. Many people come to Tai Chi later in life because of this wonderful rejuvenating aspect.

Each Tai Chi move slightly flexes a tendon, which encourages Chi to flow along the associated acupuncture meridian. The organs through which that meridian passes are energized and strengthened.

Muscles are relaxed during Tai Chi, so the flow of blood and Chi is not restricted. Where Chi goes, blood follows, so by increasing the Chi flow you boost the circulation of blood.

Each move generates centrifugal and centripetal forces which encourage the energy and blood to flow from the centre of the torso, out to the extremities, and back again, improving circulation without straining the heart.

At the higher levels of Tai Chi, special abdominal breathing exercises are introduced which not only help generate and pump Chi around the body but also massage and strengthen the internal organs.

IS TAI CHI SAFE?

Only train at your own level and always consult a teacher to make sure you are practising your Tai Chi or Chi Kung correctly. **This book is for reference only and cannot take the place of correct instruction from a competent teacher.**

As long as beginners only do beginner level techniques they will be safe. If they try intermediate techniques before they are ready, they may cause themselves some harm. If they attempt advanced level techniques they could get seriously hurt, with unbalanced physical health and mental disharmony resulting. It is important not to push the body beyond what it is comfortable doing; the aim is to train to the point of exhilaration, not exhaustion.

In many types of physical training, people say 'No pain, no gain,' and they try to 'push through' the discomfort. In Tai Chi and Chi Kung, pain is recognized as a message from the body saying that you are doing something wrong, or something needs attention. Practitioners act on the message by adjusting their posture, shifting the body weight, or increasing the Chi flow to the area to clear the stagnant energy. Alternatively, they simply stop training at that point: they are trying to build themselves up, not wear themselves down.

Tai Chi is not about having an excess of energy, but the maximum amount evenly distributed and well balanced. The aim is to feel vibrant and vitalized, not burned out. The candle that burns twice as bright burns for half as long; so tending towards moderation rather than excess ensures a longer life in better health.

In chapter 5 on Chi Kung, I explain how to balance energy in the body and store it safely in the Lower Tan Tien. If these guidelines are followed then there should be no problems with your energy or health.

Tai Chi is a lifetime's work. Progress is gradual and over a long period of time. It is not about forcing things to happen, but about training and training, and allowing them to happen when the time is right.

If the approach I have outlined in this book is followed, Tai Chi training is safe.

HOW DO I CHOOSE A TEACHER?

A good teacher should know and be able to teach the Ten Points of Correct Tai Chi Posture, the Ten Internal Principles of Tai Chi, and the Ten Methods of Practice of Tai Chi.

He should also be happy to answer any questions the students have about Tai Chi. If he has good communication skills, is able to create a good atmosphere in the class, and has a sense of humour, that is even better.

If you find a teacher with great vitality and ability, learn the techniques that he used to gain them, and develop them within yourself. A teacher is there to learn from, not to follow, so learn from him but follow yourself. A good teacher should not want people always looking to him; he should want people to look to themselves.

He may be a master of his art but he is not your master. You are your own master.

WHERE, WHEN AND FOR HOW LONG SHOULD I TRAIN?

TRAINING IN A CLASS

In a Tai Chi class, take the opportunity to train with as many different people as possible, exchange knowledge and ideas, and practise the two-person training techniques. Training with people of different heights and weights gives you the chance to develop a greater variety of responses. For example, when facing an opponent of much bigger build, you need speed and flexibility to cope with the longer reach and greater weight. If your opponent is shorter than you, he will have a lower centre of gravity, so you need to develop the ability to be rooted and stable in order not to be unbalanced by him.

Training with others increases your sensitivity to the point where on contact with an opponent, you can tell his intention. Our intention rides on our energy, which extends to the skin's surface, so when you make contact (e.g. in Push hands), your energy contacts theirs and you can read their intention.

At the most advanced level of Tai Chi, you can develop the ability to conceal your intention from the opponent, while extending your Chi field *beyond* your body, so that you can sense their intention *before* you make contact with them. These skills take many years to develop.

TRAINING ON YOUR OWN

As well as training in a class twice or three times a week, you should train by yourself every day. The benefits of Tai Chi are cumulative: it is better to do a little every day, rather than a lot one day, then nothing for a week.

Most classes are taught inside, but in your own training, take every opportunity to practise outside in natural surroundings. The fresh air and abundance of oxygen and Chi in a park or garden make it a healthier and more enjoyable place to practise Tai Chi. The quiet, calm surroundings can help you attain a deeper meditative state.

Some wonderful experiences can be had when training Tai Chi outdoors. It is possible to send your energy into the ground, like the roots of a tree, and exchange energy with the Earth. This heals both physically and spiritually.

Often, as the energy in your body increases, you see nature in a new way: the colours of the plants, flowers and trees become brighter and deeper; birdsong and the calls of other creatures become clearer. Most wonderful of all, as your energy expands and blends with the energy of the natural world, you can communicate, interact and connect with the greater spirit of nature, of which we are all a part.

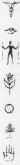

Do not train outdoors if it is too cold, hot, damp or windy, as these elemental factors can aggravate or cause illness.

WHEN SHOULD I TRAIN?

Some practitioners believe that dawn and dusk are good times to train, when the Chi is changing between Yin night and Yang day. Others say that the Yin Yang changes at midday and midnight make these good times to practise. In keeping with the Taoist philosophy of 'easy and natural is right', you can, of course, do it whenever you feel like it.

HOW LONG SHOULD I PRACTISE FOR?

The amount of time spent training each day will vary from person to person depending on their health and enthusiasm. Beginners should practise for about fifteen minutes each morning and evening; intermediate level practitioners can increase this to about half an hour twice daily; and people at an advanced level who have been training for a number of years should know their strengths and weaknesses and train for the appropriate length of time.

What you get out of Tai Chi is directly proportional to the amount of time and effort you put in.

WHAT SHOULD I WEAR?

No special clothing is required for Tai Chi: you do not need silk pyjamas or black baggy trousers. Wear what you like as long as it does not constrict your movement or blood flow. It is especially important not to wear a tight belt around your waist and belly, or a wristwatch.

If you are practising outside and it is cold, wear warm clothes to avoid catching a chill. If it is very sunny and hot, wear a hat to avoid getting heatstroke, or train in the shade.

For better posture and rooting, wear flat-soled shoes, rather than heeled or running shoes. Many people wear Chinese slippers, but I find that boating shoes are more sturdy and durable.

It is highly beneficial to practise Tai Chi barefoot on the grass so that you can draw up Earth energy through the first point on the Kidney meridian, the Bubbling Spring, on the sole of the foot.

WHAT WILL I EXPERIENCE?

People who practise Tai Chi experience Chi energy flowing through their meridians, and other Chi energy phenomena during training, sometimes separately and sometimes together.

When Chi flows round the body it feels like a warm electric glow. Aches or pains will occur where the Chi flow is blocked or stagnant: at the locations of old injuries, in areas where physical tension has built up owing to daily mental tension, or at the sites of health problems.

Whatever the causes, these areas are eventually cleared as the Chi flow increases until the whole body feels warm, healed and strong. As stagnant Chi is pushed out of the system, you may experience a dull mental nausea, but once it has cleared you will feel mentally clear and sharp.

When Chi breaks through a blocked area, mild shaking occurs, which stops when the blockage is cleared.

When the body and especially the legs start to shake more violently, this indicates complete exhaustion. If this occurs, stop training, have a big hot meal and a rest.

The third type of shaking is a humming vibration in the body, which feels like the sound a bumble bee makes and is very beneficial. It happens when the Chi is flowing smoothly through all the meridians and a person is in good health.

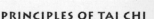

A person should only sweat either as a result of the body trying to clear heat caused by a temperature, heatstroke, or if they have been physically exerting themselves. Sweating at the beginning of a training session indicates very poor general health.

In poor health, the defensive energy on the skin's surface cannot control the pores, because it is not being supported by the internal energy which is also deficient. Spontaneous sweating indicates a need to nourish and support internal energy.

You can do this by not only training Tai Chi and Chi Kung, but by following the recommendations made in chapter 9 on Breath, by eating a lot of good healthy food, and by getting to sleep by eleven o'clock every night. If you stay up beyond this time, the body is not only being overworked, but is also being denied the time it expects to rest and recuperate. It is better to be asleep by eleven and have eight hours sleep than to go to sleep any later and get up later, because 'an hour before midnight is worth two after'.

Unexpressed emotions accumulated over time are occasionally pushed to the surface by the increased Chi flow during training. When this happens, it is best to let them out rather than suppress them again. If they are not released, they will block the Chi flow, which could lead to illness developing at a later time: it is well known that emotional and physiological pressure (stress) can cause heart attacks and stomach ulcers. If shouting or crying occur, anger and sadness are being released. When these emotions have been cleared it is not unusual to find yourself gently laughing.

The lovely healing feeling of good Chi flowing during practice can also cause spontaneous gentle laughing. This is very nice although passers-by may think you are a bit odd.

Practitioners also feel a tingling and fullness in their fingertips and other parts of the body.

When a meridian is activated you can feel its line of force through the body. At first you become more aware of the muscles, tendons and bones. Eventually Chi flows through the meridians more and more strongly, until you feel that your body is made up entirely of energy.

When you have practised for a few years, you feel as if an electromagnetic force field is building up around the hands and body.

As well as these very pleasant and enjoyable sensations, you also have a sense of weightlessness, as if in zero gravity or moving through water. At the highest level it feels as if you are made of warm, electric, liquid mercury.

WHAT ARE THE BENEFITS OF TAI CHI?

People experience a wide variety of benefits from their Tai Chi training, including: toned muscles; improved posture both when still and moving; better balance and coordination; greater self-awareness; and increased wellbeing. The stress release and relaxation response created by Tai Chi also help general health and peace of mind.

Illness is often caused by Chi stagnating in the body because of stress, poor diet or inappropriate lifestyle. Tai Chi movements encourage Chi to flow through the acupuncture meridians of the body and clear any blockages, to maintain good health.

If you suffer from cold hands and feet, they will become warmer as your circulation improves.

At the end of each training session, the energy generated is stored in the Lower Tan Tien energy centre, located just below and behind the navel. As time goes by, you accumulate more and more energy which strengthens your resistance to disease and provides a reserve which can be called upon in times of need.

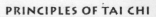

Since Tai Chi is a self-defence system, practitioners can defend themselves, their families and friends in times of danger. In peaceful times, you can enjoy the self-confidence and strengthening of spirit that comes with martial arts training.

If while practising solo forms, you imagine their self-defence applications, more energy is released because the body thinks it has more work to do. This increases energy circulation and reinforces the body's resistance. If when training the aim is to defeat your opponent, your body will apply this intention on all levels: it will also defeat harmful viruses and bacteria.

Tai Chi develops internal force (Jing): a heavy, loose, relaxed, elastic, whole body power which is different from localized, stiff, muscle power. The advantage of having Jing as part of your self-defence system is that the techniques have more power. The great force that a Tai Chi practitioner delivers is because of his Jing. It is not the arrow that kills, but the force supplied to it by the bowstring.

The body, breath, mind, emotions, energy and spirit are connected and can heal one another. Tai Chi strengthens them and brings them into harmonious balance. For example, the breath can regulate a restless mind: it is well known that to calm down, you take a deep breath and exhale through the mouth.

The increase in energy from practising Tai Chi can heal not only the body but also the emotions. Often a person with a tendency toward feeling anxious or down and lacking self-confidence has insufficient Chi energy. When you cultivate energy, you feel more substantial, confident and resilient.

If you suffer from non-specific aches and pains due to the stresses and strains of everyday life and the environment, you will find that these clear up and re-occur less, because you have more internal strength to cope with the pressures in your life and so do not get so run down.

People who do weight training say they feel very strong on the outside of their bodies, but hollow and weak inside. By training Tai Chi they become substantial and strong inside as well, because Tai Chi nourishes and strengthens not just the muscles and bones, but also the internal organs. Ultimately, the internal organs decide our strength and health.

When you have been training Tai Chi for a while, your general health will improve, you will catch colds and flu less often, get fewer aches and pains, and have a greater sense of well-being overall.

The benefits of Tai Chi result from regular practice over a long period of time. Occasionally magical things do happen but it is better to concentrate on regular daily training than to hope for a quick miracle.

To get the maximum benefit, you need to understand the Ten Points of Correct Tai Chi Posture, the Ten Internal Principles of Tai Chi, and the Ten Methods of Practice of Tai Chi. These are explained in the following chapters, so that readers who were previously only aware of Tai Chi's external appearance can familiarize themselves with its internal aspects.

I hope that you will thereby gain greater health, happiness and longevity, and make great progress on your journey of self- and spiritual development.

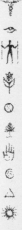

THE TEN POINTS OF CORRECT TAI CHI POSTURE

There are many different styles of Tai Chi, each of which has a slightly different emphasis. However, they all stress the importance of correct posture.

THE FEET CLAW THE GROUND

Whenever your feet make contact with the ground, claw them slightly. This helps to develop rooting and activates the first point on the Kidney meridian (K–1), through which you can exchange energy with the Earth to heal yourself and others, and make a deeper spiritual connection with nature.

By curling the toes under, you create a slight flex in the tendons. The meridians correspond to the tendons, so the flex draws the Chi down them to the toes. Remember not to hold any tension in the muscles.

THE KNEES ARE BENT

Whether you practise Tai Chi in a low or a high stance, always keep the knees slightly bent, as though you are about to sit down. Avoid putting too much stress on the knee joints by making sure that the knees are not bent further than the toes. If

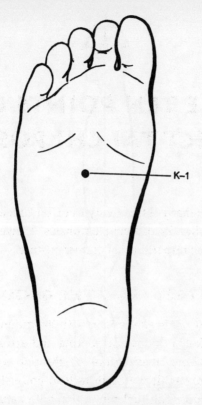

K–1

the knees pass the toes, your body weight goes into the knees; as long as they do not pass the toes, your body weight is supported by the legs, and by the feet pressing into the ground.

This position creates a slight flex in the leg tendons, which draws Chi down the corresponding meridians, ensuring a strong circulation of Chi, blood and nutrients to the legs. It also encourages the development of internal power in the legs. If your legs are strengthened, you can continue to be active in old age.

Having the knees slightly bent helps activate the Lower Tan Tien energy centre, gives you a lower centre of gravity, and greater stability.

PRINCIPLES OF TAI CHI

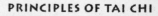

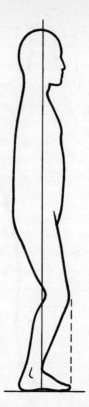

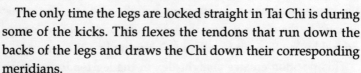

The only time the legs are locked straight in Tai Chi is during some of the kicks. This flexes the tendons that run down the backs of the legs and draws the Chi down their corresponding meridians.

The body should be aligned so that there is a vertical line between the twentieth acupuncture point on the Governing meridian (GV–20) on the top of the head, to the first acupuncture point on the Kidney meridian (K–1) on the soles of the feet.

THE ANUS SPHINCTER MUSCLE IS TENSED

There are two reasons for having the anus sphincter muscle (but not the buttocks) *slightly* tensed, pulled inward and upward. Firstly, it helps the Chi ascend up into the body, and secondly, some higher level complex internal Chi Kung exercises make use of having strength in and mental control of the anus sphincter muscle, the perineum and the sexual organs. These exercises pump the Chi and vital essence up the spine to the head.

When men have strength in and mental control over these areas, they can practise the Taoist Orgasmic Non-Ejaculatory Lovemaking Techniques which result in no Chi or essence being lost through seminal emission. Over time this conservation of Chi and essence leads to better health and greater internal power. Just prior to the loss of seminal essence, men tend to feel elated and inflated, and afterwards they feel depressed and deflated, owing to the loss of Chi and essence. The conservation of seminal essence is an important factor in maintaining not only a strong constitution but also emotional and mental stability.

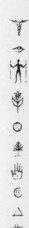

THE SPINE IS STRAIGHT
AND STRETCHED

Straightening the spine stops the edges of the vertebrae damaging the discs.

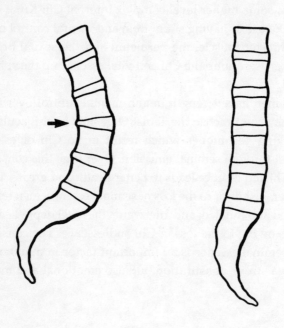

To straighten the upper spine, lift the head back and up, and
pull the chin in slightly.

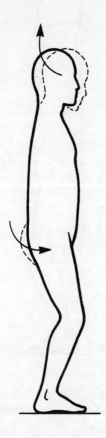

To straighten the lower spine, tilt the coccyx forward and under the torso; this should happen naturally when the knees are bent.

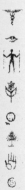

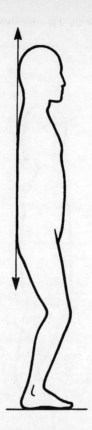

To stretch the spine along its length, imagine a string attached
to the back of the head pulling up, and a weight attached to the
lower spine pulling down.

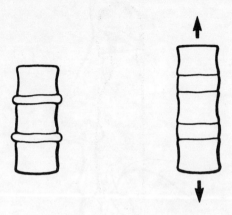

If the spine is straight and stretched while you perform the rotating, spiralling movements of Tai Chi, its flexibility is increased. The flow of spinal fluid and the function of the spinal nerves are unhindered, and Chi can ascend up the centre of the spine, through the Governing meridian, to the head.

By keeping the spine healthy, you reduce the likelihood of developing lumbago, sciatica, prolapsed discs and other back problems.

THE TONGUE IS ON
THE ROOF OF THE MOUTH

Put the tongue on the roof of the mouth at the front, just like when you say the letter L.

Keep the tongue in this position while you practise Tai Chi forms, most Chi Kung, and meditation. It allows the Chi that has risen up the Governing meridian and over the top of the head, to connect with the Conception meridian, and descend down the front of the body into the belly. This circulation of

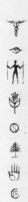

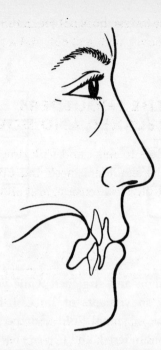

energy is commonly known as the *Small Circulation of Chi*, and with each Tai Chi move, the energy completes one orbit.

If your tongue is not connected with the roof of the mouth, energy accumulates in the head instead of travelling down to the belly. It is important never to leave excess energy in the head, because the hard bone of the skull cannot expand to take the pressure. Trapped Chi causes headaches and excessive mental activity. Neither should excess Chi be left in the chest, because the ribcage cannot expand enough, and it will cause discomfort. Only by bringing the Chi down to the belly can you be balanced and stable. The belly is soft and can expand to accommodate excess Chi: this is the safest place to store energy.

If saliva accumulates in your mouth, swallow it, as it helps carry the vital essence and energy down to the belly.

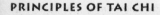

PRINCIPLES OF TAI CHI

The only times the tongue does not touch the roof are during Fa Jing explosive moves with a shout, and a few special Chi Kung exercises.

THE SHOULDERS
ARE RELAXED AND DOWN

Allow your shoulders to relax and sink down, slightly forward. This stops the shoulders, neck and upper back from storing mental and physical tension, and allows Chi to sink into the belly.

THE ELBOWS ARE
LOWER THAN THE SHOULDERS

If your elbows are below shoulder-level, it is easier for the shoulders to remain relaxed and down. If your elbow does come higher than your shoulder, as in *Crane Spreads Wings*, keep the shoulder relaxed and down: this helps the Chi to sink from the head and chest into the belly to give a lower centre of gravity.

THE ARMPITS HAVE
A SPACE UNDER THEM

You should always have a space under the armpits about the size of a fist, so that energy can flow freely through the shoulder joints and down the arms. If the undersides of the arms are touching the torso, the shoulder joint is closed and the Chi flow to the hands is reduced.

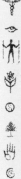

THE ARMS MAINTAIN
A CIRCULAR SHAPE

Extend the arms in front of the body, but don't quite lock the elbows. They should not be too bent, however, because this reduces the Chi flow, in the same way that bending a hosepipe stops the water from flowing. Stretch the arms forward until you feel them connected across the upper back and they form, horizontally, the shape of an archer's bow, or a horseshoe.

The arms do lock out in some of the self-defence applications, but most of the time in training they maintain this circular shape, as if you are hugging a large tree.

THE HANDS ARE
SLIGHTLY FLEXED AND CONCAVE

Flex the tendons in the hands slightly as if you are reaching out to grab someone, but relax the muscles.

The flex draws Chi down the meridians that correspond to the tendons, so you feel a fullness in your fingertips. The fingers should not be touching each other. The hands are concave so that you can hold the Chi in your palm. This posture activates the eighth point on the Pericardium meridian, which is used to emit Chi for both the martial and healing arts of Tai Chi.

Hold the thumb away from the other fingers; the web of skin between the index finger and thumb should be stretched. This activates the fourth point on the Large Intestine meridian (L1–4), which helps bring Chi from the belly and the lungs into the hands.

The martial reason for having the fingers flexed and extended is that they develop great strength with the increased Chi flow; eventually, they become like steel daggers and can be used to stab an opponent. Powerful hands and fingers capable

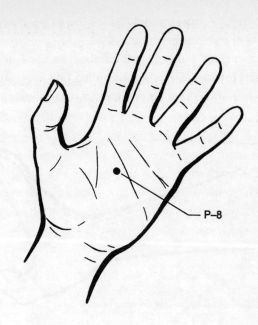

P–8

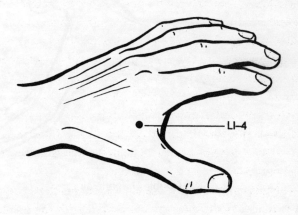

LI–4

PRINCIPLES OF TAI CHI

of emitting a concentrated flow of Chi also increase the healing effects of an acupressure massage.

The cupped palm described above is used in most Tai Chi forms. However, in the unsimplified Old Yang style, the forms also contain various other hand postures, illustrated below.

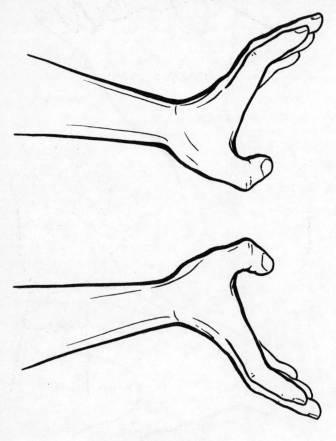

The Double Dragon Palm

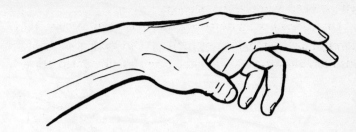

The Cobra Strike

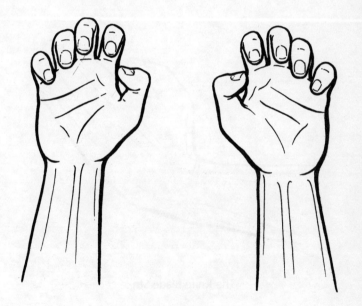

The Tiger's Claws

PRINCIPLES OF TAI CHI

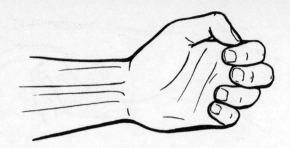

The Tiger Paw Punch

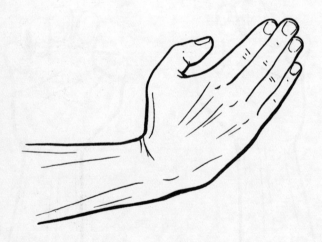

The Knife Blade Strike

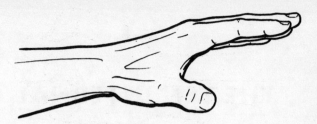

The Knife Point Strike

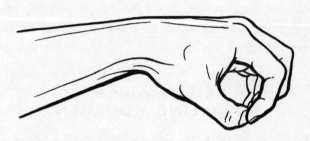

The Hook Hand

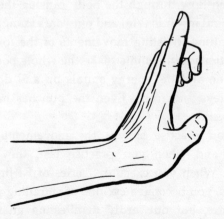

The Immortal Pointing the Way

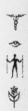

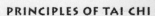

PRINCIPLES OF TAI CHI

THE TEN INTERNAL PRINCIPLES OF TAI CHI

Once you have mastered the correct posture, you can start to concentrate on some of the other internal aspects of Tai Chi.

I CIRCULAR AND SPIRALLING MOVEMENT

All Tai Chi movements are circular and spiralling. Turning the waist from side to side generates centripetal and centrifugal forces which flow through the body causing the wrists and hands to spiral inwards (Yin) and outwards (Yang).

The spiralling, twisting movements of the torso, and the subtle rotations of the joints make the whole body flow like a great river, and the energy spirals up and down around the arms, legs and torso. Even the punches have a slight corkscrew action.

When you practise slowly, the movements are like a whirlpool, and when you practise fast, they are like a whirlwind. When you execute a series of Fa Jing explosive movements, you become a cyclone of spiralling power: calm in the centre, but outwardly manifesting an unstoppable force.

Advanced practitioners can feel energy connecting the Lower Tan Tien with the diagnostic pulses of traditional Chinese medicine, located on the radial artery at the wrist.

II SLOWNESS AND SMOOTHNESS

Beginners practise Tai Chi slowly. Continuous, smooth, slow, flowing movement encourages Chi to flow in a very healing way. To develop the flow, go through the Tai Chi form once; a second time at half the speed; then a third time, at half that speed. Eventually you will be moving so slowly, with so much energy, that it will feel like walking on the moon.

Some styles of Tai Chi have Fa Jing explosive movements evenly interspersed between slow movements. This is a good way of maintaining balance in the body: slow movements are Yin, and Fa Jing movements are Yang. You move at a continuous smooth, slow, flowing rate, perform a sudden explosive Fa Jing, then move slowly and smoothly again. When movements flow, without any awkward stopping or starting, Chi flows smoothly throughout your body, balancing and healing, producing mental calm and a state of wellbeing.

By practising slowly, you enter into a meditative state, and the conscious programming of the subconscious with the Tai Chi moves and their self-defence applications is made easier. You also develop the ability to perform the moves without muscle tension, so that later you can perform them as Fa Jing effectively. If you try to Fa Jing without being relaxed, you can tear muscles.

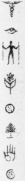

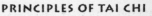

III RELAXATION AND SINKING (SUNG)

Sung means letting go of unnecessary tension in your body and mind, relaxing and sinking into the Tai Chi posture. If you let go of physical tension, it is easier to let go of mental tension, which makes it easier to let go of more physical tension, and so on. When the body is Sung, the mind can be Sung, and vice versa.

When Sung, your body becomes more supple, elastic and resilient. These youthful qualities can continue to be developed as we get older. When we are Sung there is more Chi (energy) and Jing (internal power).

In Sung, you are at ease and alert, calm and focused. When you reach out to catch a ball, you don't have to tense your muscles to be balanced and focused: it is the same with Tai Chi – your hand-eye coordination and response speed improve when you relax.

In self-defence, if you tense your muscles, they contract, and this will restrict an extending strike forward. In a relaxed state, you can extend your arm smoothly.

To achieve Sung, first let go of all tension in the shoulders, so they can sink down and slightly forward; then let go of the tensed, high-held chest, and allow it to relax and sink down – then you can let go of your clenched jaw and even smile! Next, allow your tensed, held-in belly to relax and expand; and last of all, relax the muscles in your arms and legs. It is possible to move without tension: tension just restricts the flow of blood and Chi and makes movements slow and clumsy. Though the muscles are relaxed, all the tendons in the body are slightly flexed.

Some people think a soldier has good posture: shoulders back, chest out and belly in. Sung is the opposite: shoulders forward, chest in and belly out!

All Tai Chi is done with mental intention, not muscle tension. Even at the point of impact there is no muscular tension. When Sung, your centre of gravity is lower, so that physically and mentally you are more stable and balanced. This is good for both self-defence and everyday life.

The illustrations below show the difference between a normal posture and a Sung posture.

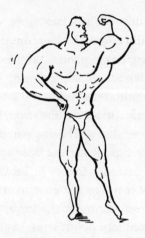

Thinks he's Mr Universe: the normal posture has a high centre of gravity and is unstable and unbalanced.

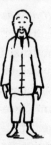

Knows he is the Universe: the Sung posture has a low centre of gravity, balance and stability.

PRINCIPLES OF TAI CHI

Rooting comes from the lower half of the body and its contact with the ground. Once this power-base has been developed, the internal force generated can be transferred to the upper body.

To develop rooting, physically sink your body weight, and imagine that it is mainly in your lower belly and legs, not in your chest and head.

Grip the ground with your feet like claws, while pushing the legs against the ground and each other. As you shift your body weight from leg to leg, one expands and the other compresses. Like springs, each leg stores and releases its coiled energy, though never one hundred per cent.

Don't let the body rise up as you shift from leg to leg, because the internal power generated will be dissipated and lost. Pushing from the legs turns the hips, waist and belly from side to side.

One of the most common stances in Tai Chi is the *Bow and Arrow*. The back foot is flat on the ground and pointing out at 45 degrees, so the toes are under the knee, giving it support and leverage. The front foot points straight ahead.

For beginners the feet are shoulder-width apart and the stance is quite long. Advanced students have a shorter, slightly narrower stance, to angle their bodies and present less of a target. They also turn their front toes inward slightly, so that the knee and leg protect the groin.

The *Bow and Arrow* stance takes its name from the appearance of the legs when the weight is forward: the front leg is bent like a bow, and the back leg looks straight like an arrow. Part of your elastic, dynamic, explosive strength comes from releasing the internal power of the legs into your arms, in the same way that a bow releases its power into an arrow. The legs always have some flex in them like a bow string, which has a flex even when it is not being drawn.

So rooting is a combination of several things: firstly, sinking the body weight into the lower body and legs by physically sinking and being Sung; secondly, clawing the ground with the feet; thirdly, pushing the leg against the ground; and fourthly, pushing the legs against each other like springs storing and releasing their power.

When these four aspects happen in conjunction with each other, you are rooted, and you can move others but remain unmoved. Rooting is the key to being the fulcrum for balance when using Tai Chi's grappling, locking, controlling and throwing techniques. For Fa Jing, you can get the power from just the waist, but by adding rooting, you have even more power.

V CENTRIFUGAL WAIST POWER

The rooting power from the Earth and the legs is controlled by the waist and belly, which turn the torso from side to side. This rotation transfers the internal force from the lower to the upper body.

Because of the weight and bulk of the waist and belly, the movement generates a great amount of centrifugal and centripetal force. Used correctly, a great amount of power can be generated in a very small space. With Fa Jing, the vigorous turn and recoil of the waist sends the hands flying out and back with explosive force.

Here is a Tai Chi warm-up technique which demonstrates this principle. Stand with your feet slightly more than shoulder-width apart, knees slightly bent, your spine straight and stretched. Keep your feet stuck to the floor, push with your left leg, and feel it turn your waist to the right. When your body weight is 70 per cent over the right leg, which has received the push from the left and feels like a compressed spring, release the coiled power by pushing with your right leg. Feel it turn

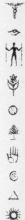

your waist round to the left until your body weight is 70 per cent over the left leg, which now compresses like a spring.

Carry on with this manoeuvre, keeping the upper body relaxed and loose as you turn from side to side, remembering to stay level. The arms are thrown outward by the centrifugal force; their movement contains great power but is totally effortless.

The combination of rooting and centrifugal waist power is devastating in combat, because you hit the opponent with not only the weight of your whole body in your hands, but also the power of your legs. The legs are three times as powerful as the arms, but the hands are three times as quick as the feet. So when you transfer the power from the legs up through the body into the hands, you have the advantage. It would be like hitting the opponent with a sledgehammer.

When incorporated into a Tai Chi form, centrifugal waist power increases the circulation of blood and Chi to the extremities without straining the heart, so improving your health.

The rotating and twisting massages all the internal organs – reservoirs of the body's energy – increasing their Chi and essence, and encouraging these to flow through the meridian system like water released from a reservoir flowing down a river.

Centrifugal and centripetal waist power is used with kicks. There are many different kicks, but the principle is the same as with the arms: the waist and belly turn back and forth and the legs are thrown out and back. So, when you kick, first the body moves, then the foot. It is the same when you execute a hand technique, like a punch or a palm strike: first the body moves, then the hand.

To develop centrifugal and centripetal waist power, go through the whole form very slowly and move the waist half a second before the rest of the body moves. Once this principle has been grasped, the hands, feet and waist appear to move at the same time.

VI UNITING THE LOWER AND UPPER BODY

A lot of power is generated by moving the lower body (hips, waist and belly) slightly ahead of the upper body (the ribcage). If the movement is disjointed, the torque power from this countermovement is lost; so don't over-emphasize it. Moving the lower body a moment before the upper body massages the thoracic diaphragm and internal organs.

When the lower and upper body are united, there is little or no time delay between the development of internal power in the legs and waist and its release from the hands.

There are three ways to help unification: firstly, position the nose directly above the navel, so that the head moves with the body; secondly, match the movement of the elbows to that of the hips, so that if the left hip bone moves forward or backward, the left elbow does too. The same applies to the right side. Thirdly and most importantly, try to keep the hands on your centre line – this is an imaginary line running down the front of the torso from the nose to the navel. If the hands ever leave this position, it should only be by a few centimetres, then they should return immediately. This is very important for self-defence Tai Chi: if your hands remain on your centre line, you can deflect your opponent's attack away from your centre as you attack his centre.

Very advanced students are taught a Chi squeezing technique, achieved by increasing and reducing the space and therefore the pressure between the ribcage and the hips. This pressure between the upper and lower body generates a compressing power which is expressed in Tai Chi's self-defence applications.

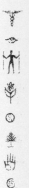

VII INTERNAL FORCE (JING)

Jing is a type of heavy, loose, relaxed, elastic whole body power which is different from localized stiff muscle power. To best understand Jing, think of the difference between an axeman chopping down a tree, and a carpenter hammering in a nail. The axeman uses his whole body in an integrated way, using his waist rotation, leg power and his arms for each stroke, whereas the carpenter uses only his arm each time he strikes.

Normal physical strength comes from the muscles expanding and contracting. Jing comes from the development of elasticity and resilience in the tendons (the connective tissue between the muscles and bones).

When you practise Tai Chi, relax the muscles in the joints, so that Chi can flow unimpeded around the body and nourish the tendons. The flex in the tendons attracts Chi; as a result they become elastic and strong. The tendons form a lattice-work from the tips of the fingers to the tips of the toes and the top of the head, and the whole body becomes a unit of dynamic, elastic power.

Jing gives Tai Chi self-defence techniques more power. The great force that a Tai Chi practitioner can deliver in his Fa Jing palm strike or punch is because of his internal force, his Jing.

The movements of people who don't let go of their muscle tension are like dead, brittle branches: if the wind blows, they break and fall down. Those who completely relax both their muscles and tendons move like limp grass that bends, and stays bent, in the wind.

In Tai Chi, you strive for balance. You don't want to be too hard (Yang) or too soft (Yin); you want to be flexible and resilient like young bamboo, so that when the wind blows, you bend, then spring back.

Jing gives you a spring in your step and a noticeable vitality to your body. As you get older you will stay flexible and active if you develop your Jing.

VIII CONNECTION

Being connected means that each part of the body is attached to and moved by a part which has moved just before, so that the rhythm of movement is like a wave through the body; with Fa Jing the movement is like a whip. The whole body moves with the flowing connection of a snake, whatever the movement. Each movement begins in the feet (which push against the ground), rises up through the legs (which push against each other), which then rotate the waist, which turns the spine, which turns the ribcage. You then feel the arm connect to the ribcage and move. The hands follow last of all. The wave-like transference of internal force through the body should be smooth and fluid.

In every Tai Chi move one connection is emphasized more than the others, but they are all still happening simultaneously. Sometimes the emphasized connection is from the right foot or leg to the right arm or hand: a same side connection (this can also be on the left). It can also be diagonal, from the right foot or leg to the left arm or hand, or from the left up to the right.

To develop connection, imagine that your whole body is moving through the air as if it were under water. Eventually your movements seem to be effortless. In beginners, the time delay as power is transferred through the body is obvious; in advanced practitioners it is not perceptible, and every part appears to move at once.

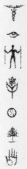

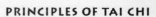

IX AVOIDING DOUBLE-WEIGHTEDNESS

The Yin-Yang balance in Tai Chi should be dynamic, otherwise the movements become double-weighted. This means that the flow is not natural, like water in a canal rather than water in a river. In Tai Chi, every part of the body is moving: your weight is constantly shifting from leg to leg, rarely evenly distributed, or fully on one leg. Usually you are shifting between having 70 per cent of your weight on one leg and 30 per cent on the other.

Never over-extend or under-extend your movements: rotate and twist in a dynamic, balanced state.

For beginners it is most important to avoid double-weightedness in the feet. Advanced practitioners are more concerned with avoiding it in the hands.

X INTEGRATION

Integration means doing the Ten Points of Correct Posture, the Ten Internal Principles, and the Ten Methods of Practice of Tai Chi at the same time. Practitioners go through a long and complex process to achieve this sensation of being made of warm, electric, liquid mercury, moving in zero gravity.

When integration is achieved, you do Tai Chi at its most advanced level. Here the emphasis is not on using your body, but your intention.

Many aspects of the Three Treasures (*see chapter 8*) become integrated: the Upper Tan Tien (thinking) with the Middle Tan Tien (feeling) and the Lower Tan Tien (doing); essence with energy and spirit; subconscious mind with conscious mind and superconscious mind; substance with function and intention; physical body with energy body and spirit body.

We all have Yin and Yang parts which need to be integrated so that our full potential can be realized. The Yin side – civilized, rational, passive and group-oriented – is used at the beginner level of Tai Chi training. The Yang side – the wild, aggressive, hunting, instinctual animal side of our nature – is only accessed at an advanced level of Tai Chi training using special techniques.

If you are only Yin and passive, you will never achieve much, but sit around and ponder this and that. By getting Yang fired up, you become mobilized and active, and take strides towards achieving your goals.

Many people are unfamiliar with and afraid of the deeper, darker, wild animal side of their nature, and some even deny its existence. Most keep it dormant, or hidden, like a wild beast locked away in the basement. Tai Chi techniques enable you to shift your awareness to a deeper part of your being, and unleash this huge reserve of untapped energy in controlled conditions, so that you slowly become familiar with it and integrate it into your overall being.

Beginners may be unaware or fearful of their Yang side; intermediate students are shown how to release it in a controlled environment, become familiar with it, and use it to achieve their objectives, without being overpowered by it. Advanced students no longer perceive themselves as having separate parts: they are not only aware of the different aspects of their being, they *are* simultaneously all the different aspects.

Ultimately in Tai Chi, the aim is to be familiar with all the different aspects of yourself; when they are unified, you are integrated.

THE TEN METHODS OF PRACTICE OF TAI CHI

The differences in how Tai Chi is practised are to do with your level of development, which I have categorized in this book as beginner, intermediate and advanced. Tai Chi has no harmful side effects when practised correctly. Never do anything to excess, but aim to make gradual progress, step by step. Never try to force things to happen; instead, relax, and let things happen in their own time. Be patient, persevere, and you will develop slowly and surely.

I STANCE

BEGINNER
Beginners have weak legs, so they start in a high stance. As their strength increases, they can make their stance lower.

INTERMEDIATE
Intermediate level practitioners using a low stance develop great strength in their legs and a lower centre of gravity, the root of power for applying Tai Chi.

At this level, practitioners have internalized their ability and can generate great internal force in the legs from an almost normal standing stance. The knees are still a little bent.

A low centre of gravity is achieved at this level by being mentally sunk into the belly and legs.

11 POSTURE

BEGINNER

Beginners concentrate on changing their S-shaped spines to straight and vertical. The upright posture creates a strong foundation for all future practice.

INTERMEDIATE

At this level, two concepts are introduced: *Lung Har Chuan* (Dragon Prawn Boxing), a way of curving the body like a prawn, or the letter C, to give greater reach when striking the opponent while hollowing out the front of the body to remain out of their range; and *Opening and Closing* (*see chapter 4*).

ADVANCED

Advanced practitioners have Lung Har Chuan and Opening and Closing in every aspect of their Tai Chi, so the posture is hunched-over because they are using the C back. This can be very confusing for beginners, who are constantly told to keep their posture upright!

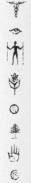

III MENTAL STATE

BEGINNER

In Tai Chi, the best way to progress is not to try and *make* things happen, but to *let* them happen. Trying to relax creates tension, you have to allow yourself to relax.

INTERMEDIATE

Intermediate level practitioners understand that Tai Chi is more experiential than intellectual. They are not in their heads, they are in their bellies: centred, balanced and calm. They are just getting on with the training and experiencing the flow and transformation of Chi within themselves. The conscious mind is no longer chattering, it is calm and quiet.

ADVANCED

Advanced level practitioners let the Tai Chi do itself. They do not have their conscious minds present to get in the way and, as a result, they have lightning reflexes.

IV BREATHING

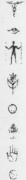

BEGINNER

Beginners keep the chest and belly relaxed and do not think about their breathing. They keep a part of their attention in the Lower Tan Tien (diagram A) in the lower belly, to help the Chi gather there.

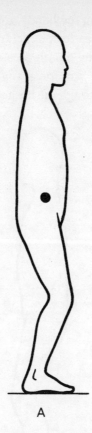

A

The Lower Tan Tien is a major energy centre. When it has accumulated, the Chi can travel from there to all other parts of the body.

INTERMEDIATE

Intermediate students use Upper Abdominal Breathing which strengthens the acquired Chi (Chi from food and air). The chest stays relaxed and down. Inhale while moving the hands down or toward the body, and allow the area between the solar plexus and the navel to expand (diagram B).

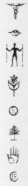

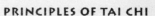

Exhale while moving the hands up or away from the body, and allow the same area to contract (diagram C). This breathing does not involve any muscle tension: it is accomplished by mental intention. Do not force anything; keep the mouth closed, and breathe through the nose slowly and calmly.

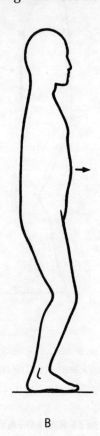

B

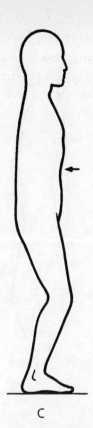

C

ADVANCED

Advanced level practitioners use Reverse Lower Abdominal breathing, which strengthens inherited Chi (the Chi you were born with). Inhale while moving the hands down or toward the body, and allow the area between the navel and the pubic bone to contract (diagram D). Exhale while moving the hands up or away from the body, and allow the same area to expand (diagram E).

Keep your mouth closed and breathe through the nose. Each breath should be calm, deep and slow, not forced but allowed to happen by itself.

PRINCIPLES OF TAI CHI

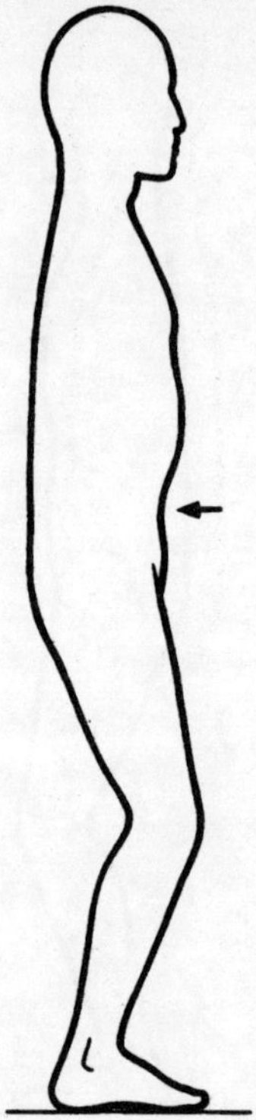

D

The body movements are totally integrated with the breathing, which should be so quiet that even you cannot hear it.

With Reverse Lower Abdominal Breathing, the kicks are done on the in-breath.

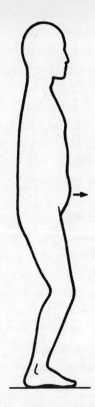

E

MOST ADVANCED

The most advanced technique is to do both Upper Abdominal Breathing and Reverse Lower Abdominal Breathing on each breath, so when you inhale with the hands moving down or toward the body, the lower abdomen moves in and the upper abdomen out. When you exhale with the hands moving up or away from the body, the lower abdomen goes out and the upper abdomen in.

PRINCIPLES OF TAI CHI

When you have been practising for some time, you will find that when you pull the lower abdomen in, you pull the sexual organs, perineum and anus up and in as well. Sedentary modern lifestyles tend to weaken the lower body, and by strengthening it you can reduce the chances of developing health problems in this area. This inward and upward activity helps to pump vital essence and Chi from the abdomen, up the centre of the spine through the Governing meridian to the head. When men have strength in and mental control over these areas, they can practise the Taoist Orgasmic Non-Ejaculatory Lovemaking Techniques.

If you inhale and hold the breath for a second before exhaling, this aids the transformation of Ching (vital essence) through Chi (vital energy) to Shen (spirit). The Chinese describe this process using the metaphor of the elements of Fire and Water. The inhalation puts the Fire (Chi from the air) below, and the Water (vital essence) above. This means that the Chi from the air is taken from the upper lungs down into the upper abdomen, and the essence from the lower abdomen is brought up into the upper abdomen, where they mix.

When you hold the breath for a second or two, the Fire heats the Water. Then, when you exhale, the Water (vital essence) returns to below (the lower abdomen) and the used-up Fire (Chi from the air) is exhaled. The steam (Chi) created by this process in the cauldron of the belly rises up through the body, healing any imbalances it encounters. When it reaches the head, it forms a fine mist (Shen), which condenses and rains back down into the cauldron of the belly, to be reheated. This replenishing of the essence in the cauldron of the belly is encouraged by storing the Chi in the Lower Tan Tien when you finish training. The process continues and, over time, the spirit becomes purified and substantial. A bigger spirit means a stronger will, greater creativity and an expanded awareness.

Keep the belly relaxed and don't think about the breathing.

V EYES

BEGINNERS

When doing the solo forms, beginners watch the horizon with a calm expression. This helps keep your head upright and allows you to relax.

Occasionally doing the whole form with your eyes closed helps to develop internal balance and improve your sense of direction.

INTERMEDIATE

When doing the solo forms, intermediate level practitioners watch the hand that is doing the main part of the application. This helps lead the Chi to the hands because the eyes and intention are linked, and Chi energy follows intention.

This use of focus vision connects your movements with your conscious mind. If during training you visualize yourself applying the moves against imaginary opponents, you are consciously programming them into your subconscious.

There are many techniques for healing other people using your energy, or by allowing universal energy to flow through you, out of your hands, and into the patient. To get good results from energy healing (also known as External Chi Kung healing), you must be able to lead the energy accurately into the relevant acupuncture points and along the appropriate meridians in the patient. Your eyes can be used to focus your intention to lead the energy where it needs to go.

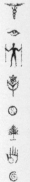

ADVANCED

At this level, move the eyes so that the hands are always in the area of your peripheral vision. Peripheral vision connects with the subconscious mind and this has two benefits.

Firstly, because the subconscious is activated and thinks that you really are going to do the martial applications of Tai Chi, a great amount of Chi is released. Because you are not using this Chi against an opponent, it rushes around your body, healing imbalances and improving your health.

Secondly, when applying Tai Chi in self-defence, because the subconscious has been programmed with all the Tai Chi moves and applications, and is several hundred times faster at responding than the conscious mind, you have a greater chance of defeating the opponent. By keeping the opponent or opponents in your peripheral field of view, any offensive movement made toward you immediately triggers a subconscious response.

In most life-and-death situations, if you were to waste valuable seconds consciously thinking of which response to use, it would probably be too late.

By understanding the connection between the eyes, energy and intention, you can develop your martial arts and healing skills to a very high level.

MOST ADVANCED

At this level a system called *Da Mo's Eyes* is used. The Chi released with this system has a wild, uncivilized quality; its use results in an extreme state of increased Chi, heightened awareness, and the activation of survival instincts. It takes some time to return to a calmer state.

Da Mo's Eyes allows you to access vast amounts of Chi instantly, and to expand your field of perception. It helps to develop 'feeling with the Chi' (*see chapter 8*).

It is also a way to tap Yang emotional states, and to channel that raw, emotionally charged Chi into your movements and their self-defence applications.

The technique should only be taught to a practitioner who is emotionally well-balanced with great self-knowledge, and a strong sense of justice and honour.

VI HAND CIRCLES AND WAIST ROTATION

BEGINNER

Beginners should make large, expressive hand circles and waist rotations, to release physical and mental tension and open up their meridians.

The waist moves first, then a split second later the hands move. This is so that the centrifugal and centripetal waist power is correctly transferred to the hands.

INTERMEDIATE

Intermediate students have learned how to let go of physical and mental tension, so they no longer need such expansive movements, and can make their waist rotations and corresponding hand circles smaller. They have less external physical movement and more internal energetic movement.

ADVANCED

The waist turns from side to side, and the hands are thrown out and back. When the right hip bone moves forward the right elbow moves forward. When the waist rotates the other way and the right hip bone moves back, the right elbow follows. The same relationship exists between the left elbow and hip.

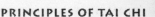

MOST ADVANCED

At this very high level an additional hip movement is introduced into every Tai Chi posture, to a greater or lesser degree. Like many other high level techniques it is very subtle and cannot easily be seen by an outside observer.

To develop this body rocking technique, observe the self-defence application of each posture, then move so that your hips provide the power for it.

At less advanced levels the hips move backward and forward, now they also rock diagonally up and down.

For example, if you have your right foot forward while doing an uppercut punch with your right hand, your fist begins from your lower right side and travels diagonally up and across a little toward your left. You will hit the opponent in his left floating rib. Instead of just rotating your waist to the left as you bring your body weight forward onto your right foot, you also subtly rock the hips. You tilt the right hip down a bit, then up, as you bring your body weight forward onto the right leg. So the rising right elbow is being pushed upward by the rising right hip. The upward strike, done as a Fa Jing, has your body weight and waist rotating power behind it.

This example uses one application to convey the advanced body rocking movement. All Tai Chi postures have several applications, so the hips rock diagonally up and down, as well as forward and backward several times in each move.

If you strike diagonally up, from left to right or right to left, there is one type of hip rocking; if you strike diagonally down, there is another.

As with all aspects of Tai Chi, a practitioner needs to be shown this by a capable teacher.

VII FA JING
– AN EXPLOSIVE MOVEMENT

BEGINNER

Beginners do not practise Fa Jing. They practise doing the Tai Chi moves slowly, without muscle tension, to build up their Chi. You can only Fa Jing when you have no muscle tension in the body.

INTERMEDIATE

Intermediate students begin tentatively to practise Fa Jing as a conscious action.

To Fa Jing, vigorously shake your waist; the shake travels through the whole body. By the time it reaches the hands and feet the force is concentrated, so your punch or kick has great power.

The Fa Jing concentrated shaking force is similar in many ways to cracking a bullwhip: the movement of the handle is not that fast but by the time the flowing force has reached the end of the whip it is travelling at over six hundred miles per hour, faster than the speed of sound.

Part of the supersonic cracking sound when the end of the whip flicks is caused by the pull-back on the handle of the whip. The usual whip handle motion is up and down and up again suddenly. This creates a wave that flows along the whip and causes the tip to flick and crack.

When you Fa Jing with your body it is the same: the waist turns out, back, and out again suddenly. The waist shake sends a wave along the body, out to the hands which flick and snap.

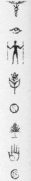

Advanced Fa Jing moves are done with the Ten Points of Correct Tai Chi Posture, the Ten Internal Principles of Tai Chi and the advanced level aspects of the Ten Methods of Practice of Tai Chi.

Advanced level practitioners do Fa Jing in all the different areas of Tai Chi. They have an excess of Chi that they need to release, and can throw themselves into Fa Jing. Big Fa Jing throw the whole body forward a complete step. Small Fa Jing cause the body to shuffle forward a little.

At an advanced level, your conscious mind is not present when you Fa Jing, just like when you sneeze. Often, the release of Chi is so great that you get 'blown away' – you temporarily lose your sense of self. Then you become aware of your body again, and carry on with the Tai Chi. During the time that you are 'gone', great healing can occur because you are not 'there' to get in the way.

At an advanced level this phenomenon occurs not just on Fa Jing moves but during the whole form. You remember starting the form, and finishing it, but you were not 'there' during the half hour it took you to do the form.

Fa Jing is a vigorous whole body shaking force during which you exhale, push the lower abdomen out and vigorously turn the waist so that the hands are thrown out while you shout 'BA!' or 'PA!' (the B or P helps store the energy and the A helps to release it). The recoil of the waist takes you into the next Fa Jing. Very advanced practitioners can create their own sounds for their Fa Jing movements. The Fa Jing generates so much expanding energy that the shout becomes necessary to release it.

When using Fa Jing in combat, the shout has an adverse effect on the opponent, and exhaling stops you from being winded if you take a blow. Your internal organs are protected by the expansion of your belly, which also releases the Chi into the rest of the body so powerfully that your counterstrike has unstoppable force.

In training, Fa Jing has great healing power, and in the martial applications of Tai Chi it has a devastating effect on the opponent.

Tai Chi's slow movements build up the Chi, and Fa Jing explosive movements release the excess. Slow movements without Fa Jing are like Yin without Yang: unbalanced.

When you practise the slow movements your energy wave is long:

When you do a Fa Jing it is short:

When you change from one to the other, there is no break in your movements because they are all part of the same Chi flow:

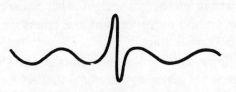

At an advanced level, every Fa Jing is done with an Opening or Closing movement at the same time.

Intermediate students have one self-defence application on each Fa Jing movement: advanced students have two or three.

In combat you can Fa Jing to strike not only with the fists and feet but also the knees, elbows, shoulders and head. Whichever part of your body is closest to the opponent becomes the weapon you use to strike a target area on his body.

MOST ADVANCED

When you have been practising for a number of years your Fa Jing movements become more internalized. Although the actual physical movement is smaller, the explosive release of internal force is greater. The shout has more power but less volume.

At this stage, small, shaking Fa Jing movements start to happen spontaneously on almost every Tai Chi move.

At the highest level of Fa Jing self-defence training, you aim to hit specific acupuncture points on the opponent's body. Depending on how and which point you hit, you can cause different things to happen to the opponent, such as disorientation, collapse and unconsciousness.

To adversely affect the opponent's Chi via his acupuncture points, each point must be struck in a specific way: either upward or downward; inward or outward spiralling; left to right or right to left; toward or away from yourself; diagonal up or down from left to right or right to left. Some of the above are done while you move forward and others while moving backward (reverse Fa Jing).

With Fa Jing counterstrikes, the points must be hit in a specific sequence, for example, you might first contact points on the opponent's arms or legs, then their torso or head.

When these advanced aspects of the Fa Jing have been mastered, with the Chi of your counterstrike, you can disorientate

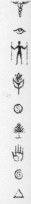

the opponent by scattering their Chi, or drain their energy,
causing them to collapse from weakness.

You can temporarily paralyse parts of the opponent's body by blocking his Chi flow, and cause unconsciousness by directing the Fa Jing's shocking power through the meridian system into vital organs and body systems.

If your life and the lives of friends and family are threatened, and there is no alternative, you can use the Chi of your Fa Jing to stop the Chi flow in the opponent's body permanently.

VIII OPENING AND CLOSING

BEGINNER

Beginners do not include special breathing in their training.

INTERMEDIATE

Intermediate students are told which moves are Open and which are Closed but the technique is not fully explained to them. They use Upper Abdominal Breathing in their Tai Chi.

ADVANCED

Advanced level practitioners use Reverse Lower Abdominal Breathing and are shown how to use Opening and Closing with each Tai Chi move. Opening and Closing is breathing not just with the belly, but with the whole body. They are small, internal movements not perceptible to an observer.

To Open and Close means to bend and straighten the two bows of the body in conjunction with Reverse Lower Abdominal Breathing.

The Horizontal Arm Bow is a line from the tip of your middle finger, up the outside of the arm, across the back, and down the outside of the other arm to the tip of the middle finger on the other hand. The Vertical Spine Bow is a single line from the coccyx up the spine to the crown of the head.

When the bows are straight, the hands apart, the spine straight and the breath and the lower belly in, you are Opening. When the bows are bent, the hands slightly closer together, the spine curved like a crescent moon, and the breath and lower belly out, you are Closing.

When Closing, do not make the mistake of breaking the horizontal arm bow at the shoulders as if you were carrying a box. The arms, back muscles and shoulder blades come close to the spine when you Open and all move away from the spine as you Close.

Before doing the form, practise Opening and Closing in the Basic Chi Kung Standing Posture to build up the energy between the palms.

Opening and Closing at an advanced level is achieved by a specific type of pressure on the insides of the knees, as if there were a spring between the legs pushing the knees outward.

Opening and Closing the feet helps your rooting to the ground, and to pump the healing Earth Chi up into the body through acupuncture point Kidney–1 (the Bubbling Spring).

In each movement as you finish Closing, you are already Opening, and vice versa. This is because Tai Chi contains Yin in Yang and Yang in Yin in constant flux.

At a very advanced level students learn how to Open on one side of the body while Closing on the other.

When you are Closed the spine is in the shape of the letter C. The C back releases great Yang energy from the spine into the rest of the body, which increases your instinctive survival awareness.

BEGINNER

Beginners concentrate on the Yin Yang changes in the legs: storing and releasing internal power, and shifting the body weight – from leg to leg.

INTERMEDIATE

Intermediate students concentrate on the Yin Yang change of the waist turning from side to side. The centrifugal and centripetal waist power is a result of the push from the legs: the leg pushes, the waist turns, the hand is thrown out to hit the target. You do not punch through the target, nor do you punch and stop on impact: the centrifugal Yang and centripetal Yin energies mean that you punch and pull back to give a penetrating, percussive blow to the opponent. This Yin-Yang waist recoil action can happen independently of the leg power.

ADVANCED

Advanced practitioners use the Yin and Yang changes of the legs, waist and Opening and Closing movements.

The most advanced Yin Yang change is in the hands: a continual flow between a Yang palm and a Yin palm. Neither are ever one hundred per cent Yin or Yang; there is always transformation from one to the other. When the forearm moves up, the hand trails behind slightly so that it points down a little. When the forearm moves down, the hand trails behind slightly so that it points up a little. This is the vertical Yin Yang palm change.

The horizontal Yin Yang palm change happens when the forearm moves to the right and the hand trails behind slightly so that it points to the left, and when the forearm moves to the left, so the hand trails slightly behind and points to the right.

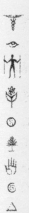

This flowing change makes the hands look as if they are trailing through water, or like the wings of a large bird.

In Tai Chi, nothing is linear, because you are always turning, rotating and twisting, so the hands and wrists do not move simply horizontally or vertically but in inward spirals (Yin) and outward spirals (Yang).

The Yin-Yang palm changes store and release Chi. As the hand releases its Yang Chi it accumulates Yin Chi, and vice versa.

As your ability develops, a very powerful Chi density builds up in and around the hands, which feels like an electromagnetic force field.

X INTERNALIZATION

BEGINNER

Beginners concentrate on internalizing the Ten Points of Correct Tai Chi Posture, so that they can go from being in their normal posture to being in the Tai Chi posture without appearing to have changed in any way. This is useful because if you find yourself in a potentially violent situation, you want to be ready to respond, but you do not want to provoke an attack by making an obvious offensive movement. Tai Chi's fighting stance looks like a normal standing stance.

INTERMEDIATE

Intermediate students concentrate on internalizing the Ten Internal Principles and the Ten Methods of Practice of Tai Chi. You use all these abilities which are now under your subconscious control, and do not have to be consciously initiated. Only an experienced observer can tell what you are doing. A passer-by might notice that there was something going on but would not be able to say what it was.

At this level, things happen that are hard to convey and are best understood by personally experiencing them. You are no longer just your body or your Chi, your subconscious or your conscious: you are also your superconscious – your spirit.

The Tai Chi is done with intention (*see chapter 8*).

By becoming so internalized you trigger an equal and opposite occurrence, and your spirit is externalized: you are inside and outside yourself at the same time, and can shift your awareness to your spirit body.

At this level you attain the Wu Chi way of perceiving the world. The Tai Chi way of perceiving is the normal, everyday reality – the physical world – where everything is dualistic: there is always a subject–object relationship in which things are judged as good or bad, and time is linear.

When you perceive the Wu Chi way, there is no duality, no subject or object, because you realize how everything is part of everything else. Good and bad are no longer fixed, they fluctuate as circumstances change. Time is no longer a one way journey: the relationship between the past, present and future changes in the most mysterious and interesting ways.

Tai Chi is the Yin-Yang diagram; Wu Chi is symbolized by an empty circle.

To be balanced, a Tai Chi practitioner must be comfortable and confident in both realities. He must be able to move from one to the other at will, and to exist in both simultaneously.

Tai Chi and Wu Chi flow into one another and together comprise the Tao (the Way, *see chapter 11*). Each person is Tai Chi and Wu Chi simultaneously: each person is Tao.

CHI KUNG

Chi Kung means exercises that work with energy, so Tai Chi is a type of Chi Kung.

In this chapter two Chi Kung exercises are explained, which are often practised alongside and within Tai Chi: the *Basic Chi Kung Standing Posture* (also known as the *Universal Posture*, *Three Circle Chi Kung* or the *Embracing the Tree Posture*); and the *Small Circulation of Chi* (also known as *The Small Heavenly Circle* or *The Microcosmic Orbit*). Both complement Tai Chi training and help to increase energy, improve health, and balance the mind and emotions. They are usually practised before a training session as a warm up and afterwards as a cool down, but can also be practised independently (*see chapter 1*, What will I experience?).

THE BASIC CHI KUNG STANDING POSTURE

To do the Basic Chi Kung Standing Posture, stand with your feet a little more than shoulder-width apart, your body weight *slightly* more on the heels than the toes, and your hands in front of you as if hugging a large tree. Use the Ten Points of Correct Posture, keep the hands at the shoulder-height, and be Sung, so that greater amounts of Chi can flow and more Jing can be developed.

Beginners hold the posture for two minutes, and add ten seconds each day until they get up to five minutes. Intermediate students extend this to about ten minutes, and advanced students should know their strengths and weaknesses, and choose the appropriate length of time accordingly.

The posture activates the Chi in the Lower Tan Tien and releases it into the body so that it reaches the ends of the fingers and toes and the top of the head. You will experience Chi energy flowing through the meridians like a warm electric glow. When a meridian is activated you can feel its line of force through the body. You may also feel a tingling and fullness in the fingertips and other parts of the body.

THE SMALL CIRCULATION OF CHI

The Small Circulation of Chi takes the Chi from the Lower Tan Tien, under the torso, up the spine through the Governing meridian, over the top of the head and then down the front of the body along the Conception meridian and back into the Lower Tan Tien. The circuit becomes more and more open the longer you practise Tai Chi and Chi Kung. The Governing and Conception meridians can store more Chi than any other meridian, and circulating the Chi through them helps to fill them up.

The Chi is led through the Small Circulation by your intention: your strength of will takes the Chi from point to point around the body. Although you can use breathing to help move Chi, you should not be dependent on it. When you have been practising for some time the channels open fully and the Chi flows freely through them almost effortlessly. It makes one full circulation in each Tai Chi movement.

The Small Circulation of Chi is most often practised in the Basic Chi Kung Standing Posture but it can also be practised while sitting down. In the Basic Chi Kung Standing Posture, begin by smiling down to the Lower Tan Tien to activate your energy with a positive intention. Try to clear your mind of thoughts. If you can't, think positive things.

When you feel Chi in the Lower Tan Tien, bring it forward to C–6, the Ocean of Chi (see diagram opposite). (In acupuncture, this point is used to replenish the vital essence and increase Chi.) Lead it through the Sexual Palace C–4, the sexual organs, the perineum C–1, the anus sphincter muscle and G–1 at the coccyx.

Then take it up through the centre of the spine along G–4, G–6, G–11, G–14, G–16 in the occipital cavity and G–20 on the top of the head (through which you can absorb universal healing energy), then to the third eye (between the eyebrows), through the roof of the mouth to the tip of the tongue, down to the throat C–22, the chest C–17, the solar plexus C–12, the navel C–8, back to C–6, and from there back to the Lower Tan Tien.

This is one circuit. To do more, instead of going from C–6 back to the Lower Tan Tien, continue straight on to the Sexual Palace and go round the circuit again, only returning to the Lower Tan Tien when you have done your final circuit.

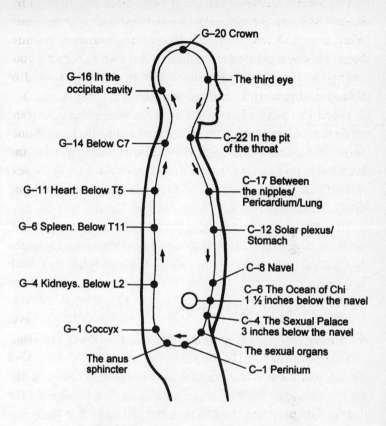

G–20 Crown

G–16 In the occipital cavity

The third eye

G–14 Below C7

C–22 In the pit of the throat

G–11 Heart. Below T5

C–17 Between the nipples/ Pericardium/Lung

G–6 Spleen. Below T11

C–12 Solar plexus/ Stomach

C–8 Navel

G–4 Kidneys. Below L2

C–6 The Ocean of Chi 1 ½ inches below the navel

C–4 The Sexual Palace 3 inches below the navel

G–1 Coccyx

The sexual organs

The anus sphincter

C–1 Perinium

G= Governing Meridian, runs up the centre of the back
C= Conception Meridian, runs along the mid-line of the
    front of the body

C7= Cervical vertebrae number seven
T5= Thoracic vertebrae number five
T11= Thoracic vertebrae number eleven
L2= Lumbar vertebrae number two

The Small Circulation of Chi

PRINCIPLES OF TAI CHI

Having completed three, six or nine orbits of the Small Circulation of Chi, store the Chi in the Lower Tan Tien by placing the palms over C–6, the Ocean of Chi, and concentrating on it while rubbing it gently for a minute.

When the Chi is in the Lower Tan Tien, the belly might expand slightly, or feel more substantial. This pleasant sensation produces a calm, happy feeling and a warmth in your centre. At this point, think positive things, like 'I feel powerful and peaceful, balanced and calm deep down inside myself.' Or don't think, just be.

The Small Circulation of Chi helps to transform of Ching (vital essence) to Chi (vital energy) to Shen (spirit), and ensures that the Chi is more evenly distributed around the body.

Always finish Tai Chi, Chi Kung or meditation by bringing the Chi back to the Lower Tan Tien and storing it there.

WHEN WILL I DO CHI KUNG?

A training session incorporating the two Chi Kung exercises described is structured in the following way.

First, you spend a few minutes in the Basic Chi Kung Standing Posture, and do three, six or nine circuits of the Small Circulation of Chi, bring the Chi back to the Lower Tan Tien, not to store it but to centre yourself.

Now that the energy is activated you do your Tai Chi training: single and two-person forms, weapons, etc. Afterwards, you spend a few minutes in the Basic Chi Kung Standing Posture, and do three, six or nine circuits of the Small Circulation of Chi, then store the Chi you have generated in the Lower Tan Tien. Often, any excess energy radiates from the hands as a warm glow.

This excess in the hands can be used for self-healing: for example, place the palms of your hands over your kidneys while leaning forward a little. Breathe in and expand the kidneys, then as you breathe out, you send the warm, healing Chi from the palms of your hands, into the kidneys. Repeat this a few times until the kidneys feel warm and full.

According to Traditional Chinese Medicine the kidneys are among the most important organs in the body. Great care should be taken of them because so many other organs and body systems depend on their good health.

Over time, you gradually accumulate more and more Chi energy, which can be used to heal yourself and others; to enhance whatever activities you channel it into; and to bring about positive changes in your life. If you are full of Chi you tend to be more cheerful.

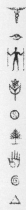

6

TAI CHI
WEAPONS FORMS

The weapons forms are usually taught when the empty hand forms have been learnt. They contain the Ten Points of Correct Posture, the Ten Internal Principles, and the Ten Methods of Practice of Tai Chi.

Tai Chi has several weapons forms, including the *Long Sword and Dagger*, the *Single Sabre* and *Double Sabre*, the *Short Stick*, *Staff* and *Spear*. The *Walking Stick* form is very useful for old people living in dangerous places, because they can have a weapon to defend themselves with, which is legal and does not attract attention.

Traditionally, in the Sword and Dagger form, the sword is held in the right hand and the dagger in the left. Most people today no longer use the dagger, so the left hand is empty.

The Double Sabre form exercises both sides of the body. (With the other weapons forms, first you learn them with the weapon in the right hand, then in the left.)

Some people believe that the sabre – a variation on the machette – was the first weapon, that the Single Sabre form was the first weapons form, and so should be learnt first. Others claim that the short stick was man's first tool, the Short Stick was the first form, and so should be learnt first.

In general, the short single weapons are taught first: Short Stick, Walking Stick, and Single Sabre. The double weapons forms come next: Double Sabre and the Sword and Dagger; and last are the long weapons forms, the Staff and the Spear.

All the weapons eventually feel as if they are a part of you, like an extra limb, and the Chi that emanates from you extends to the end of the weapon.

All the weapons forms at an advanced level contain Fa Jing. The walking stick must be made of rattan, which is flexible, so that the Fa Jing shaking energy can flow to the end of the weapon. If the wooden weapon is hard and stiff, the shaking Chi can get trapped in the body and cause damage.

When practising the weapons forms you must be Sung. The body releases more Chi to support the extra weight you are holding, and the increased Chi flowing round the body results in greater healing.

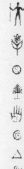

TAI CHI
FIGHTING STRATEGY

RESPONSES

YIN RESPONSE TO A YIN SITUATION

In a Yin situation, there is very little chance of getting seriously hurt, for example, if the opponent is very weak, drunk and cannot coordinate his movements. Use a Yin response – any one of Tai Chi's huge array of controlling manoeuvres – to subdue the opponent, or a pushing or pulling technique to throw him away.

YANG RESPONSE TO A YANG SITUATION

In a Yang situation, the opponent or opponents have every intention of seriously injuring or killing you. A Yang response is to use Fa Jing counterstrikes with the intention of stopping the opponent immediately.

YANG RESPONSE TO A YIN SITUATION

To use a Yang response in a Yin situation is unvirtuous. There is no benefit in such an act: causing unnecessary harm to others harms yourself. Only use Tai Chi's Yang responses when you have no choice.

To use a Yin response in a Yang situation may be thought of as correct moral behaviour, but the advantage it gives the opponent may lead to your own defeat. Only a practitioner who has reached the peak of his ability should consider using a Yin response in a Yang situation.

TAI CHI FIGHTING STANCE

The Tai Chi fighting stance looks like a normal standing stance, but internally all the correct Points of Posture, Internal Principles and Methods of Practice of Tai Chi have been automatically activated by your subconscious at the first hint of danger.

The Tai Chi fighting stance does not provoke the opponent unnecessarily, which increases the chances of avoiding a confrontation. If your opponent makes the mistake of attacking you, you are ready to respond to any move.

HOW TO USE THE FOUR DIRECTIONS AND FOUR CORNERS

Imagine you are standing in the middle of a compass, with North straight ahead, South behind, West to the left, and East to the right. These are the Four Directions.

Diagonally forward to the left is northwest, diagonally forward to the right is northeast, diagonally back to the left is southwest and diagonally back to the right is southeast. These are the Four Corners.

When an opponent attacks you, depending on his angle of attack, you step into one of the Four Corners or Four Directions.

There are so many combinations it would be impossible to list them all, so I will only give a few examples to convey the basic idea.

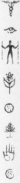

If your opponent attacks you head on but you have a greater body weight than he, and you are able to generate more Yang offensive energy, Fa Jing to the north straight into him.

If he has a greater body weight and his attack appears to be ferocious, step back into the southeast or southwest corners while you Fa Jing attack him. This way you avoid the full force of his attack.

When you apply Tai Chi in combat, northeast or northwest are the directions most often used. This is so you can generate offensive energy by moving forward with your Fa Jing into the opponent, and avoid the full force of his attack by stepping to the northeast or northwest.

WINDOWS AND DOORS

Windows and Doors are metaphors for ways of getting through the opponent's defensive perimeter. For example, if he steps forward with his right foot and throws a straight right punch, you Fa Jing step forward with your left foot to the northwest, and your waist rotates to the right. The back (right) foot is moved slightly to the West by the force of the Fa Jing.

The Fa Jing centrifugal power of the waist rotation to the right throws the arms upward and out: at this point you are Opening.

As you start to Close, your right hand hits the outside of your opponent's arm just above his right elbow, either to deflect the attacking arm, or damage the elbow. The final part of the Closing is when the left hand a split second later hits either his head or exposed ribs. Using this Door is a good way in.

You must seize the windows of opportunity created by the opponent's attack and end the confrontation decisively and immediately. This allows you to be ready to face any accomplices the opponent may have with him.

THE THREE DISTANCES

The use of the Eight Directions and Windows and Doors is possible if you know how to use the Three Distances.

The first distance is Outside: here you are beyond the opponent's punching and kicking distance.

Next is the Middle, where your and the opponent's limbs can impact with each other, but you are not close enough to hit his torso or his head.

The last one is Inside: you are so close to him that you can hit his torso and head.

If you stay Outside, the opponent cannot reach you. If he should make the mistake of attacking, thus giving you a Door, move as he moves and step through the Door. While passing through the Middle you control and deflect the opponent off your centre line and place yourself in a position to attack. Once you are Inside, strike repeatedly and decisively.

CODE OF VIRTUOUS MARTIAL CONDUCT – TAI CHI VERSION

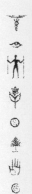

- Never attack first, because you do not want to open any Windows or Doors for the opponent to get Inside. Wait for him to make his offensive move, and as soon as he does, or you sense their intention to do so, counterattack.

- Tai Chi is for defence: when someone attacks you, defend yourself, using only the appropriate Yin or Yang response.

- Do not start fights and avoid known trouble spots: you are training to build yourself up rather than to bring others down.

- Train and train every day, but aim never to use Tai Chi in combat. If you become involved in a confrontation, try every possible means of avoiding a fight.

So if you practise Tai Chi but never use it for self-defence, what is the point? Well, by practising Tai Chi daily, you end up being very healthy, happy and having a long life!

CODE OF VIRTUOUS MARTIAL CONDUCT – WU CHI VERSION

The Tai Chi way of perceiving life in which there is Yin and Yang duality, subject and object, you and the opponent, the 'us and them' attitude, which promotes confrontation, is only half of the picture.

When you perceive the Wu Chi way, you realize that all things are interconnected. This understanding promotes compassion instead of confrontation.

Sometimes you have to use force to resolve situations, but really there is no enemy out there. There are just situations that need to be resolved. If a person is having thoughts of verbal or physical conflict with another, it is likely that they have unresolved conflicts within themselves.

THE THREE TREASURES

The Three Treasures have many strands, which intertwine to produce a tapestry of understanding about how our internal worlds and the external world relate to one another. All three exist simultaneously, integrated and continually transforming into one another. They can be divided into the following categories:

Physical World • Energy World • Spirit World

Ching (vital essence) • Chi (vital energy) •* Shen (spirit)

Conscious Mind • Subconscious Mind • Superconscious Mind

Substance • Function • Intention

Physical Body • Energy Body • Spirit Body

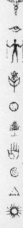

THE THREE TREASURES OF THE PHYSICAL WORLD, THE ENERGY WORLD AND THE SPIRIT WORLD

Some people are only comfortable with the modern world of cars, fast food, television and materialism. Others shun everyday life and devote themselves to the mysterious and ancient spirit world. The third way is not to see everyday life and spirituality as opposites, but to embrace both at the same time.

All the worlds overlap and interact, and are part of one another. A person is also a composite of spirit, energy and a physical body. When you realize this, the possibilities in your life open up and you are no longer limited by the laws of physical mechanics because you can tap into energy dynamics and vast spiritual forces.

Your connection with the physical world is through the senses that you were encouraged to develop in a certain way as children. It is possible to activate dormant senses through Tai Chi training, so that you perceive and experience the energy and spirit worlds. These dormant senses do not have universally accepted names and it is very hard to convey to someone who has not experienced them what they are like. If in a dream you see a new colour, when you wake up, how do you describe it to someone?

The first dormant sense usually awakened by Tai Chi's two-person training exercises could be called 'seeing with the skin'. When your eyes are closed and you make contact with an opponent, you can still 'see' where he is and what he intends to do.

The next dormant sense to awaken could be called 'feeling with Chi', which means that you can feel your opponent with your energy and know his intention, although you have not made physical contact with him.

By experiencing and understanding the world of Chi inside you through the practice of Tai Chi and Chi Kung, it becomes possible to feel and interact with the Chi of other people.

When you heal a person with energy flowing through you into them, you give it a positive intention by being Sung and maintaining a healing feeling. You need to be able to generate this Sung healing feeling in your own Tai Chi training for self-healing before you can heal others.

When you become more familiar with your energy and spirit, you can sense the energy and spirit of the land, trees, plants and animals, and communicate with them.

If you are Sung in a forest or other natural place, you can see Chi around the trees, around yourself and other people. It is vibrant glow shimmering in the air. (There is more Chi in forests than in cities, which have more busy activity but less natural energy.)

Everything is alive because, like us, everything is composed of a combination of physical substance, energetic activity and spirit: everything is connected to everything else physically, energetically and spiritually. When you throw a stone into a pond, the ripples spread outwards. It is the same with everything we think, feel, say and do: they all have an effect on the worlds around us, especially if there is a strong intention to them.

Tai Chi and Chi Kung develop various natural abilities that we all have to a greater or lesser degree, for example, the ability to see energy, people who are no longer in their bodies, and non-human spirit entities, and the ability to channel energy through yourself to heal others. (Universal Healing Chi is absorbed through GV–20 at the top of the head, and Earth Chi is absorbed through K–1 on the soles of the feet. These combined energies are emitted through the palms of the hands via P–8 into the patient.) Telepathy, enhanced intuition,

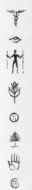

empathy and knowledge of the immediate future, all become more easily attainable.

It is very important that these natural abilities are only used to help and heal others. If you use them to control, manipulate or harm, then because of the dynamics of universal balance, you will be setting in motion a series of events that will eventually harm yourself.

THE THREE TREASURES OF VITAL ESSENCE, VITAL ENERGY AND SPIRIT

According to ancient Taoist theory there are three treasures within the body: Ching (vital essence), Chi (vital energy) and Shen (spirit).

When you practise Tai Chi, you transform vital essence into vital energy into spirit. The process of using up our essence (Ching) to give ourselves a functional power (Chi) so that we can carry out our intentions (Shen) is a natural one. It can be described symbolically in the following way.

Imagine a cauldron in the belly containing your Ching, the Elixir of Life. When the cauldron is heated, steam rises and permeates the whole body. The steam is Chi energy. On reaching the head, it condenses and rains back down into the cauldron in the belly to be reheated.

When this process has been happening for a while, a very fine vapour like energy collects in the head. This is Shen.

The higher the level of Tai Chi, the more the processes of transformation and circulation are activated. Fa Jing movements are particularly effective in causing an internal vapourization of the vital essence: it is like lifting the lid of a boiling pot to let off some steam.

In old age, when less vital essence remains in the body, it can become like a tree with no sap. The bones become like brittle

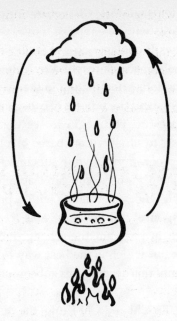

branches and the skin like dead leaves. If you conserve your vital essence and train Tai Chi every day, then even in old age you will have a supple, resilient body, and remain healthy and active with a sound mind and strong spirit.

THE THREE TREASURES OF THE SUBCONSCIOUS, CONSCIOUS AND SUPERCONSCIOUS MINDS

The subconscious mind carries out various automatic functions and can store huge amounts of information. When you practise Tai Chi, and notice that your posture or hand-eye coordination is incorrect, you continually, consciously correct it. Eventually your posture is corrected and your hand-eye coordination improves. This is because you have consciously reprogrammed your subconscious.

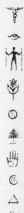

PRINCIPLES OF TAI CHI

You can go on to program it with various response actions. If an opponent attacks with one type of move, you can counter-attack with another. If you ever do use Tai Chi for self-defence, you can let the subconscious respond quickly and effectively, without your conscious mind getting in the way.

When you understand the process of consciously reprogramming the subconscious, you begin to see that some of your everyday responses to situations are based on old subconscious programs. By reprogramming your subconscious with more sensible, up-to-date responses, you can lead a happier life. For example, a person who, when faced with a problem, has the subconscious response, 'I'll never be able to work this out', should first notice the program, then change it by continuously saying, 'I'll work out which is the best way to deal with this, and then do it!' until this becomes his subconscious response to all problems.

While training Tai Chi and Chi Kung, the door between the conscious and subconscious is more open than usual, so it is a good time to reprogram the subconscious with positive intentions.

Old patterns of behaviour and unresolved issues trap energy, which can be freed again for us to use. While clearing an issue, you may find emotions associated with it that have never been expressed. These need to be released: the suppressed emotion is an energy block which if left might lead to illness developing.

For many people the change caused by clearing an old issue is a frightening leap into the unknown, but a person on the path of self-development is always looking to clear away limitations in order to enjoy more freedom, with increased energy, greater mental clarity and improved health.

Training strengthens your spirit, and you become more able to set a strong intention to move forward on your journey of self-development. When you get to the traumatic emotional stage in the process of clearing an old issue, instead of turning back, you carry on because you know the reward of breaking through to the other side is worth pursuing.

There is an old Taoist saying, 'Eradicate the negative and develop the positive.' It means that we should get illness out of the body and keep it out, remove unhealthy attitudes and develop positive ones.

Tai Chi calms the usually agitated conscious mind. This is the meditative aspect of Tai Chi that many people are familiar with. Don't *try* to meditate while doing Tai Chi: if you are doing it correctly, it just happens.

When the conscious mind is calm, mental and physical tension is released. Beginners use this relaxation response to release stress that they have accumulated during the day. Advanced practitioners doing Tai Chi's full contact two-person training exercises remain mentally and physically Sung – relaxed but dynamic and aware, even though they are under great pressure. They take this ability into everyday life so they can work under pressure and not accumulate stress.

When the conscious mind is calm enough, enlightening insights from the superconscious can manifest themselves. If you practise Tai Chi regularly, you will spontaneously experience moments of deep insight and clarity in everyday life. Sometimes your visual perception might change: colours become more intense, angles sharpen, and you see patterns in previously random things. At other times, insight results in great creative work or the solution to a problem. Eventually, the superconscious mind becomes a tangible voice in your head, giving clear, wise advice. As time goes by, all three minds become a single, clear, awareness.

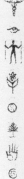

THE THREE TREASURES OF SUBSTANCE, FUNCTION AND INTENTION

The substance of the physical body has its functional activity powered by energy, and intention is the spiritual force that initiates everything.

Ice is a solid which can transform into liquid water, and into steam which can rise up into the sky. Ice, water and steam are the same thing in different states; a person is much the same in relation to substance, function and intention.

In advanced Tai Chi training, you move in such a way that your body seems to melt and flow, and your spirit can ascend out of your body and you can look down at yourself doing Tai Chi. This is accomplished by doing Tai Chi with your intention.

Intention is a spiritual force that must be cultivated if you are to achieve your highest objectives. The substance of your physical body is like the size of a sword, your energy is its momentum (functional strength), and your intention is the sharpness of the blade.

This level is above all previously mentioned in this book. You need to have been practising Tai Chi and Chi Kung for many years and be totally proficient at the most advanced levels of the Ten Points of Correct Tai Chi Posture, the Ten Internal Principles of Tai Chi, and the Ten Methods of Practice of Tai Chi.

Lead your spirit body with your intention, and your physical body follows. Once you have done the move with the spirit, there is no need to repeat it with the physical body, so you go on to the next move: you do less with your physical body and more with your spirit body. Do the whole form in this way.

The internal development of your intention eventually enables you to externalize your spirit, and you watch from a slightly elevated position as your physical body goes through the Tai Chi form.

After many years of practice, you feel as familiar with your spirit body as you do with your physical body, and are able to fly in your spirit body as naturally as walking in your physical body. (Separation from the physical body sometimes happens when you are asleep, under anaesthetic or have been knocked out. Many people have had these out-of-body experiences or very vivid dreams of falling or flying.)

At the time of death we must permanently leave our physical bodies. At a very advanced level of Tai Chi, the transition into spirit is familiar and the spirit world is a place you have visited many times, so you are able to enjoyably continue your journey of development and discovery in the great unlimited cosmos.

THE THREE TREASURES OF THE PHYSICAL BODY, THE ENERGY BODY AND THE SPIRITUAL BODY

It is possible to strengthen your physical body so that it lasts long enough to develop an energy body, which can be transformed into an immortal spirit body. To attain this spiritual immortality, it is important to have a sensible lifestyle, a healthy diet and to practise Tai Chi and Chi Kung daily.

Understanding the Chi energy inside yourself is the key to unlocking the door to the spirit world. First, use your energy to strengthen your physical body, then fill up all the organs, Tan Tiens, and acupuncture meridians with Chi. Refine your Ching essence into Chi energy into Shen spirit, and use the spiritual energy to nourish and cultivate the spirit body inside you.

When you are ready, 'open the door' on the top of your head and rise up out of yourself into the spirit world.

To understand the complexity of the spirit world, consider the physical world: there is land, air and sea which are all inhabited by a wide variety of different creatures. There are different races of people, and people with different opinions and attitudes. The spirit world is just as varied, complicated and interesting.

By becoming familiar with the idea of existing outside your physical body, the fear of death is overcome. Knowing that death is not the end, but just a change of state, allows you to enjoy life more.

Spiritual immortality takes a lifetime to achieve.

One of the most inspiring descriptions of out-of-body travel is by the 18th century Taoist adept, Liu I Ming in his book *Awakening to the Tao*.

Transformations of a Spiritual Dragon

A dragon as a spiritual luminosity can be large or small; it can rise and descend, disappear and appear, penetrate rocks and mountains, leap in the clouds and travel with the rain. How can it do all this? It is done by the activity of the spirit.

What I realise as I observe this is the Tao of inconceivable spiritual transmutation. The reason humans can be humans is because of the spirit. As long as the spirit is there, they live. When the spirit leaves, they die.

The spirit penetrates heaven and Earth, knows the past and present, enters into every subtlety, and exists in every place. It enters water without drowning, fire without burning, penetrates metal and rock without hindrance. It is so large that it fills the universe, so small that it fits into a hairtip. It is imperceptible, ungraspable, inexplicable, indescribable.

One who can use the spirit skilfully changes in accordance with the times and therefore can share the qualities of heaven and earth, the light of the sun and the moon, the order of the four seasons; command nature in the primordial state; and serve nature in the temporal state. This is like the transformations of a spiritual dragon, which cannot be seen in the traces of form.

TAKEN FROM *AWAKENING THE TAO* BY TAO-LIU I-MING,

TRANSLATED BY THOMAS CLEARY (SHAMBALA PUBLICATIONS)

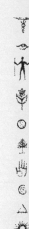

BREATH, EMOTIONS AND TWO-PERSON EXERCISES

Your breathing changes during your life. In the womb you use Reverse Abdominal Breathing, pulling in the lower belly to draw in energy from your mother through the umbilical cord, and expanding it to send waste out. When you are born, for the first few years of your life you use Deep Abdominal Breathing.

In middle age, you tend to breathe from the chest; in old age, you wheeze from the upper chest, and at the point of death a final breath comes from the throat, there is one last shallow exhalation through the mouth and nose, and you are gone.

The nearer to death you get, the higher and thinner your breathing becomes, so by making your breathing deep and full, you can continually rejuvenate yourself and enjoy a longer and healthier life.

Most people's breathing is controlled by their subconscious mind, and is a reflection of their health. Unhealthy people become breathless after a small amount of exercise. With Tai Chi training, you gain conscious control of your breathing and use it to improve your health. Special breathing techniques are used which enable greater amounts of the Chi and oxygen from the air to be absorbed into your system. Instead of being breathless, you are Chi-full.

When people breathe normally, it is usually just with their chests. This uses just half of the lung capacity. It is better to use the lungs to full capacity, to increase the oxygenation of the blood and the amount of external Chi taken deeper into the body.

To accomplish this, make your normal breathing long, slow, calm and deep. When you inhale, expand not only your chest, but your upper and lower abdomen. When you exhale, allow the upper and lower abdomen to contract. The movement of the upper and lower abdomen in and out is no more than an inch. Use this breathing for normal activities during the day.

When you do Tai Chi at an intermediate level, use Upper Abdominal Breathing: inhale, expand the chest a little, but the upper abdomen – the area between the solar plexus and the navel – much more. This expands the lungs to their fullest capacity. When you exhale, pull the upper abdomen in to empty the lungs and make them ready to inhale fresh air. Upper Abdominal Breathing promotes digestion, absorption and circulation.

At a more advanced level, use Reverse Lower Abdominal Breathing. This does not interfere with the Upper Abdominal Breathing and has many benefits. When you inhale, pull in the lower abdomen – the area between the navel and the pubic bone – and when you exhale, expand the area. This type of breathing strengthens urination, defecation and reproduction, and helps to create vital essence and distribute it around the body.

Both types of breathing massage and strengthen the internal organs and strengthen inspiration and expiration.

By pumping the body up and increasing the amount of Chi you have inside pushing out, you increase your body's resistance to viruses, bacteria and adverse weather conditions. Strong internal energy strengthens your defensive energy.

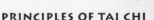

PRINCIPLES OF TAI CHI

Whichever type of breathing you are doing, as you inhale and exhale, the energy moves through the Small Circulation of Chi.

On the inhalation, Upper Abdominal Breathing takes the Chi mainly down the Conception meridian and only a little up the Governing meridian. On the exhalation, Chi goes mainly up the Governing meridian and only a little down the Conception meridian.

With Reverse Lower Abdominal Breathing, it is the other way round. When you inhale, Chi goes mainly up the back through the Governing meridian, and only a little down the Conception meridian. When you exhale, it goes mainly down the Conception meridian and only a little up the Governing meridian.

The Chi also flows through a variety of other meridians as it goes from the Lower Tan Tien out to the hands, feet and head and back again, in conjunction with exhilation and inhalation.

When you are at a high level, every now and then, practise the form without paying any attention to the breathing at all. Relax the belly as you flow through the moves.

After a few years, once you have consciously programmed these breathing techniques into the subconscious, you will find that they happen by themselves, even when you are not doing Tai Chi.

They can also be used to regulate your mind and emotions: there is a strong connection between the breath, the mind and emotions. For example, when a person gets angry he tends to hold his breath, and when he gets anxious and panics, his breath tends to become shorter and shallower.

People who don't practise any form of breathing exercises find that when they arrive in a difficult situation these responses can result in a lack of mental clarity and a wrong decision.

In a high pressure situation, you must either intentionally temporarily suppress your emotions and deal with the situation, or, if appropriate, intentionally express your emotions, put your Chi into them, and use them to help you resolve the situation.

In a social situation the expression of emotions is verbal; in a self-defence situation they are released physically through the Fa Jing. In training the Fa Jing can be used as an intentional emotional release.

There is no rule about when to suppress or express emotions. The important thing is to be familiar with them, so that they are a help rather than a hindrance when trying to resolve a situation.

So if you can consciously control your breath and get it to work for you, you can regulate your emotions, keep a clear mind and make the right decisions.

Here is a simple example of how to use your breathing to help regain your balance when you are too angry, anxious or fearful. This technique is for when it is not beneficial or appropriate for you to express your emotions. Inhale a deep breath through your nose and exhale through your mouth slowly several times. This calms the system and enables you to think more clearly.

There are occasions when it is very beneficial to let your emotions flow. If a person is experiencing grief, expressing it through crying is a release. Staring without blinking is a way to induce crying. If a person experiences great anger, shouting helps to release it.

If it is not appropriate to express the emotion at the time, it is vital to release it later. An emotion rising up to be released is a movement of Chi: if it is suppressed, the Chi flow is blocked, and this can lead to illness developing.

So as well as talking things through to clear the mind, you also have to clear the suppressed emotions from the body. When the trapped emotions have cleared there is easy laughter.

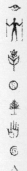

After training Tai Chi and Chi Kung for a few years you find that you can be calm, breathe easily and be focused in circumstances that previously would have made you uncontrollably emotional. Instead of being ruled by your emotions you can get them to work for you. Emotions are neither good nor bad, but a help or a hindrance depending on circumstance. Sometimes they are there when you don't need them and not there when you do!

If you bring the emotions under the control of your conscious mind, you can use their energy to help achieve your objectives. For example, when an opponent is about to attack, you experience a combination of fear and anger, both of which release vast amounts of energy into your system. If you know how, you can channel this emotionally generated energy through your Fa Jing. Otherwise, the emotions can be overwhelming and result in you freezing to the spot or succumbing to irrational behaviour.

The two-person training techniques when done with Fa Jing enable you to experience something close to the intensity of real combat with the emotions that it generates.

They also help develop a more powerful type of Jing internal force. This is like the process for making a good sword blade: the metal is repeatedly heated, folded, hammered and allowed to cool. The Chi released is the heating, the pressure experienced from the incoming force of the opponent is the folding. The full contact aspect of the self-defence application is the hammering, and Chi Kung is the cooling.

Beginners do not use much forward pressure when practising the two-person systems; they concentrate on developing more sensitivity. Advanced practitioners use considerable forward pressure to develop upper body power and whole body Jing.

There are many two-person training exercises: Pushing Hands, Da Lu and Lung Har Chuan (Dragon Prawn Boxing) are a few well known examples. In the Old Yang style of Tai Chi there is the San Sau Two-Person Fighting form which contains full contact explosive Fa Jing counterstrikes all the way through.

The New Yang style of Tai Chi has simplified the San Sau, which emphasizes the idea of stepping backward as the opponent advances, then stepping forward as he retreats; in the Old Yang style, when he advances, you advance with your counterstrike.

All types of two-person training exercises give you a greater understanding of timing, distance, and increase your sensitivity to other people's energy, which is beneficial for self-defence and healing others.

TAO

The beauty of the Way is that there is no Way.

LOY CHING-YUEN

Tao literally means 'The Way', however, because it is an abstract idea, each person has their own interpretation of it.

For some people, to follow the Tao means to be in tune with the natural world. To others, it is about maintaining a healthy balance in their lives: mentally, emotionally, energetically, physically, spiritually and socially. Some perceive Tao as their spirit, or the spirit of the universe. These people aim to follow Tao and be Tao.

Tao cannot be defined simply, because we are all different, and we must each follow our own path through life, our own Way.

I hope that the information contained in this book will be a small contribution to your life's journey, and help to bring you a greater ability in self-defence, improve your health and well-being and enhance your self- and spiritual development.

RESOURCES

There are many good teachers who are not part of any school or association.

To find out where Tai Chi is taught, look in the alternative health advertising sections of local papers or listings magazines, and at the back of martial arts magazines. Many sports centres and health clubs offer Tai Chi classes, so ring them to see what is available.

If there are a few places to learn Tai Chi nearby, watch or join in a class at each place before you choose.

THE WORLD TAIJI
BOXING ASSOCIATION

The World Taiji Boxing Association has its headquarters in Australia and members in 35 different countries. As well as having qualified instructors it has an information centre called MTG Publishing which produces over 100 videos on all aspects of the internal martial arts and a quarterly magazine called *Combat and Healing*.

WTBA INSTRUCTORS IN THE UNITED KINGDOM

For information about WTBA instructors in the north of England, call:
Ian Watts – 0161 766 1668

For information about WTBA instructors in Wales, call:
Peter Jones – 01792 898721

MTG Publishing has a branch in Wales. For a catalogue call:
Tony Court – 01792 418808

For information about WTBA instructors in the east of England, call:
Colin Orr – 01493 601111

For information about WTBA instructors in southeast England, call:
Jim Uglow – 0836 665509

For information about WTBA instructors in London, call:
Paul Brecher – 0181 264 8074

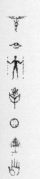

Master Erle Montaigue has been the Head of the World Taiji Boxing Association since 1984. He is world famous for his Taiji-quan (Tai Chi Chuan), Qigong (Chi Kung) and Bagwa (Pa Kwa), and holds regular workshops in New South Wales. To find out about WTBA instructors in your part of Australia or New Zealand and to receive a WTBA catalogue, write to Erle at:

PO Box 792
Murwillumbah
NSW 2484
Australia

http://www.ozmail.com.au/taiji/

WTBA INSTRUCTORS IN THE USA

Alexander Krych is the Chief WTBA instructor in the USA. He has trained under some of the world's greatest instructors and has attained a high level of training and teaching. Al teaches most of the Erle Montaigue system and hosts his USA work-shops. To find out about WTBA instructors in your part of the USA, write to Al at:

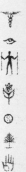

c/o Belvidere Post Office
Belvidere
New Jersey
07823–2018
USA

Tel: 908 475 1619
E-mail: 74640.2154@compuserve.com

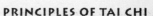

Mike Babin is the Chief Instructor in Canada for the WTBA. He teaches Bagwa (Pa Kwa), Qigong (Chi Kung), Taijiquan (Tai Chi Chuan), and most of the Erle Montaigue system. Like Al Krych, Michael is one of the nicest people you are likely to meet and be lucky enough to have as an instructor. Mike teaches in Ottawa and hosts Erle's workshops in Canada. To find out about WTBA instructors in your part of Canada, write to Mike at:

Tai Chi Studio WTBA
195A Bank Street
2nd Floor
Ottawa
Ontario
K2P1W7
Canada

Tel: 613 235 3493
E-mail: lois@globalx.net

ABOUT THE AUTHOR

At a high level of skill the practitioner has pride over his ability, rejoices in praise from others, and laments the lack of ability in others. At the highest level, a man has the look of knowing nothing.

ANCIENT TAOIST WISDOM

Paul Brecher has over twenty years of experience in the martial arts and is an Instructor of the World Tai Chi Boxing Association. He has written numerous articles for magazines and given Tai Chi demonstrations on television.

In his London classes he teaches Yang Lu Chan's Old Yang Style Tai Chi Long Form, The Old Yang Style Tai Chi San Sau Two-Person Fighting Form, The Old Yang Style Pauchui Cannon Fist Form, and Tai Chi Weapons Forms: Double Sabre, Staff, Walking Stick. He also teaches Pushing Hands, Da Lu, Tai Chi Lung Har Chuan (Dragon Prawn Boxing), Three Circle Chi Kung, the Small Circulation and Large Circulation of Chi, Iron Shirt and Iron Palm Chi Kung, and the Twelve Circular Tai Chi Dim Mak Palms.

As well as being involved with the martial arts, he is a practitioner of Traditional Chinese Medicine.

Paul Brecher BA MAcS MPCHM (Bachelor of Arts, Member of the Acupuncture Society, and Member Practitioner of

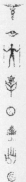

Chinese Herbal Medicine) can be contacted at the following address:

PO BOX 13219
London NW11 7WS

Tel: 0181 264 8074

PRINCIPLES OF ACUPUNCTURE

ANGELA HICKS

Acupuncture is a Chinese therapy who efficacy is well known in the Western medical community. It has been proved effective in treating a wide range of conditions from asthma to high blood pressure. This book provides anyone contemplating a useful overview of acupuncture and the principles of Chinese medicine including:

- how diagnosis is made in Chinese medicine

- which illnesses acupuncture treats effectively

- how the needles are used and how they affect your body systems

- how to find a practitioner.

Angela Hicks qualified as an acupuncturist in 1976. She is co-principal of the College of Integrated Chinese Medicine, and she lectures in the UK and the USA.

PRINCIPLES OF CHINESE MEDICINE

ANGELA HICKS

Acupuncture, Chinese herbs, Qigong, Tui Na massage and diet therapy have been used by the Chinese for over 2,000 years, and they are still the treatments of choice for millions of people throughout the East. Now, despite the availability of Western medicine, Westerners are becoming aware of the many benefits of these potent therapies and the popularity of Chinese medicine is spreading rapidly.

This introductory guide contains:

- the basic theory of Chinese medicine
- an account of traditional Chinese diagnosis and each of the five therapies
- patients' first-hand accounts of their treatment
- how to find a practitioner.

Angela Hicks qualified as an acupuncturist in 1976. She is co-principal of the College of Integrated Chinese Medicine, and she lectures in the UK and the USA.

PRINCIPLES OF
CHINESE HERBAL MEDICINE

JOHN HICKS

China has a 5,000 year-old tradition of herbal medicine. In this book, John Hicks explains the system and lists the most popular and effective herbs, roots, fruits and seeds and what health conditions they can treat. With this accessible and informative guide you will also learn:

- how Chinese herbal medicine can work in tandem with Western medical diagnosis

- what symptoms can be treated – from eczema to digestive troubles

- how to find a practitioner.

John Hicks is the founder and co-principal of the College of Integrated Chinese Medicine. He has been a practising acupuncturist, Chinese herbalist and teacher for over 15 years.

PRINCIPLES OF FENG SHUI

SIMON BROWN

Feng Shui is the ancient Oriental system of organizing your home and workplace in a way that promotes health, happiness and success. Learning the basic principles can help you transform your environment. This introductory guide explains:

- what Feng Shui is and how it works

- simple, practical ways of finding the best possible placement for objects, furniture and rooms

- how to find your personal Feng Shui number and calculate the best timing, when travelling or making changes in your home and workplace

- how to find which direction is best for you, for sleeping, working and optimizing your energy and creativity

- what to expect from a professional Feng Shui consultant.

Principles of Acupuncture	0 7225 3409 4	£5.99	☐
Principles of Chinese Medicine	0 7225 3215 6	£5.99	☐
Principles of Chinese Herbal Medicine	0 7225 3341 1	£5.99	☐
Principles of Feng Shui	0 7225 3347 0	£5.99	☐

All these books are available from your local bookseller or can be ordered direct from the publishers.

To order direct just tick the titles you want and fill in the form below:

Name: _____

Address: _____

_____

_____ Postcode: _____

Send to Thorsons Mail Order, Dept 3, HarperCollins*Publishers*, Westerhill Road, Bishopbriggs, Glasgow G64 2QT.
Please enclose a cheque or postal order or your authority to debit your Visa/Access account —

Credit card no: _____

Expiry date: _____

Signature: _____

— up to the value of the cover price plus:
UK & BFPO: Add £1.00 for the first book and 25p for each additional book ordered.

Overseas orders including Eire: Please add £2.95 service charge. Books will be sent by surface mail but quotes for airmail dispatches will be given on request.

24-HOUR TELEPHONE ORDERING SERVICE FOR ACCESS/VISA CARDHOLDERS — TEL: 0141 772 2281.